DENTAL MANAGEMENT OF SYSTEMIC DISORDERS: A CLINICAL HANDBOOK

Dr Swapnil Chincholikar,
Dr Aarti Goel

notionpress.com

INDIA · SINGAPORE · MALAYSIA

ISBN
Paperback 979-8-90479-604-4
Hardcase 979-8-90479-605-1

Dedication

This book is dedicated to patients, who have been our greatest teachers. Their trust, resilience, and diverse clinical challenges have continually inspired us to deepen our understanding of the intricate relationship between systemic and oral health.

We also dedicate this work to our mentors and teachers, whose guidance, wisdom, and encouragement has shaped our clinical thinking and professional journey.

Finally, to our parents and family, for their unwavering support, patience, and belief in us throughout this endeavour.

Contents

Acknowledgement

We express our sincere and heartfelt gratitude to all those who have supported and guided us in the successful completion of this book.

We humbly acknowledge the blessings of the Almighty, our parents, Dr SM Chincholikar, Dr Nilima Chincholikar, Mr Sudip Goel, Mrs Bindu Goel and our family, Ms Parul Goel, whose grace has enabled us to undertake and accomplish this work. Their faith in us has been a constant source of strength.

We are deeply indebted to our respected teachers and mentors Dr. J. Sridevi, Dr Shankar Iyer, Dr Kirpa Johar for their constant encouragement, invaluable guidance, and clinical wisdom, which has played a pivotal role in shaping this work.

We extend our sincere thanks to our friend Dr Anmol Kapoor, for his insightful discussions and constructive suggestions.

We would also like to acknowledge our patients, whose diverse clinical conditions and trust in our care has provided invaluable learning experiences and practical insights into the dental management of systemic disorders.

Finally, We are thankful to the publisher and editorial team for their cooperation, patience, and assistance in bringing this work to completion.

Place: Bangalore

Date : 15.04.2026

Dr Swapnil Chincholikar

Dr Aarti Goel

Foreword

Modern dental practice has evolved significantly, with clinicians increasingly managing an aging population presenting with multiple comorbidities, alongside younger patients affected by lifestyle-related systemic conditions. Contemporary dentistry therefore demands a comprehensive, patient-centered approach that extends beyond oral health alone.

A thorough understanding of systemic diseases, ongoing medical therapies, and potential drug interactions is essential for delivering safe and effective dental care. Clinical decision-making must take into account the patient's overall medical status, including the need to modify, defer, or appropriately plan treatment to minimize risks and prevent complications.

This handbook on the dental management of systemic disorders serves as a practical and accessible reference for clinicians. Its structured format enables quick retrieval of essential information and provides evidence-based modifications to treatment protocols where necessary. By bridging the disciplines of medicine and dentistry, it supports safer practice and improved patient outcomes.

I strongly recommend this handbook to both experienced clinicians and emerging practitioners. It will serve as a valuable guide in ensuring patient safety and maintaining high standards of clinical care.

The authors are to be commended for presenting complex medical concepts in a clear, concise, and clinically relevant manner.

Dr. J. Sridevi, M.D.S.

Private Practitioner

Ex Professor & HOD, Dept Of Prosthodontics,

DAPMRV Dental College & Hospital,

Bangalore

Preface

Dentistry in India has changed significantly over the last few decades. As clinicians, we now routinely treat patients who are living longer, managing multiple medical conditions, and taking several medications on a long-term basis. If you have been in dental practice for even a few years, you already know this reality: most patients walking into our clinics today come with more than just a dental complaint. Diabetes, hypertension, heart disease, asthma, thyroid problems, kidney issues, long-term medications and so-on.

Almost all of us have faced moments of doubt at the chairside. *Can I safely do this extraction? How much local anesthesia is okay for this patient? Should I ask for a medical fitness? Should I defer the treatment/what blood tests should I ask the patient to do?* In many cases, the problem is not lack of willingness to treat, but lack of clear, practical guidance that applies to day-to-day dental practice.

This book has been written keeping those exact situations in mind. It does not aim to turn dentists into physicians, nor does it overload the reader with unnecessary medical details. Instead, it focuses on what dentists really need to know—how a systemic condition affects dental treatment, what precautions are essential, when to proceed, when to modify treatment, and when to refer.

The approach throughout this book is simple and practical. Each chapter discusses a systemic disorder from a dental point of view, highlighting common clinical scenarios, drug considerations, and safety measures.

This book is meant for practicing dentists, postgraduate students, and specialists who want to feel more confident while treating medically compromised patients. It is designed to be a quick reference as well as a learning guide—something you can turn to before starting a procedure, or even when planning treatment for a complex patient.

At the end of the day, dentistry is not just about teeth—it is about treating people. Understanding their medical background allows us to provide safer, better, and more responsible care. If this handbook helps reduce hesitation, improves confidence, and supports safer clinical practice, then it has achieved its purpose.

Chapter 1

Dental Management of Patients with Gastrointestinal Disorders

Introduction

Many gastrointestinal diseases present with oral symptoms that are detectable by dentists and often, oral manifestations of the disease may appear before systemic signs and symptoms. Managing patients with these conditions requires dentists to adjust their treatment and/or involve other health professionals and take consent from the gastroenterologist.

Care must be taken when providing periodontal therapy or dental implants to patients suffering from gastrointestinal diseases who are at high risk of bleeding, infection, or malnutrition. Also, pharmacological therapy for these patients needs to be customized.

1. Pepticulcer & GERD

Table 1-1: Dental considerations in Peptic ulcer & GERD

Aspect	Clinical Considerations for Dentists
Local anaesthesia & epinephrine	No specific precautions or contraindications with epinephrine in patients taking antacids, H2-receptor antagonists, or proton pump inhibitors (PPIs).
Drug–drug interactions	Always review potential drug interactions with medications commonly prescribed for PUD/GERD before prescribing dental drugs.
Antibiotic prescription	Patients may already be on amoxicillin and clarithromycin for *H. pylori* therapy. Do not increase the dose or repeat the same antibiotics. Prescribe an antibiotic from a different class (e.g., clindamycin), if indicated.
NSAID use	Actively ask about OTC and prescription NSAIDs (e.g., ibuprofen, diclofenac, naproxen). Avoid prescribing NSAIDs in patients with a current or past history of PUD or severe GERD. Prefer paracetamol for pain control.
Steroid prescription	Avoid systemic corticosteroids in patients with peptic ulcer disease, as they may aggravate gastric mucosal injury.
OTC medications	Specifically ask about OTC drugs, as many ulcer and GERD medications are available without prescription (e.g., antacids, cimetidine, omeprazole).
Tetracyclines & antacids	In patients taking only antacids, tetracycline or doxycycline should not be taken concurrently. Maintain a 1–2-hour gap to avoid reduced antibiotic absorption.
Black hairy tongue	May occur with antacids, bismuth subsalicylate, and tetracycline. Reassure patients that this is temporary and resolves after stopping the medication.

Aspect	**Clinical Considerations for Dentists**
Oral manifestations of GERD	GERD may present with burning mouth sensation, tooth erosion, and hypersensitivity. GERD should be considered as a differential diagnosis for burning mouth symptoms.
Dental chair position	Treat patients in a semi-supine position rather than fully supine to reduce reflux and discomfort.
Acid neutralization	Recommend sodium bicarbonate (Baking soda) mouthrinse after reflux episodes to help neutralize oral acidity.
Preventive dental care	Apply in-office topical fluoride and consider prescribing home-applied fluoride for patients with chronic GERD to reduce erosion and sensitivity. (Rehabilitation with composite/ceramic restorations in advanced cases)

2. Irritable Bowel Syndrome

Table 1-2: Dental considerations in Irritable Bowel Syndrome

Dental Drug Prescribed	**Interacting Drug (IBS/GI)**	**Clinical Effect**	**Management for Dentist**
Paracetamol + hydrocodone/ codeine/ oxycodone	Bismuth subsalicylate	Increased blood levels and adverse effects of the dental drug; may cause severe abdominal cramps or bloating	Use with caution or substitute with another analgesic (prefer paracetamol alone if possible)
Doxycycline, Tetracycline	Bismuth subsalicylate	Decreased absorption and reduced efficacy of the antibiotic	Separate doses by 2–3 hours
Penicillin	Cholestyramine	Reduced absorption of penicillin	Separate doses by 1–2 hours

(Contd.)

Dental Drug Prescribed	Interacting Drug (IBS/GI)	Clinical Effect	Management for Dentist
Epinephrine in local anaesthetic	Tricyclic antidepressants (TCAs)	Increased synaptic levels of epinephrine and norepinephrine → risk of hypertension and cardiac arrhythmias	Epinephrine not contraindicated, but limit dose to max 2 cartridges of 1:80,000
Levonordefrin (in LA)	Tricyclic antidepressants (TCAs)	Marked hypertensive response	CONTRAINDICATED – do not use
Epinephrine in local anaesthetic	SSRIs	No significant interaction	Safe to use

3. Crohns Disease

Table 1-3: Dental considerations in Crohn's Disease

Category	Considerations	Recommendations
1. **Steroid Use & Periodontal Health**	Corticosteroids (e.g., Prednisone) may induce steroid-related diabetes → ↑ periodontal disease risk	• Monitor periodontal status closely • Maintain strict oral hygiene • Epinephrine in local anaesthesia generally safe
2. **Immunosuppressive Therapy – Cyclosporine**	Cyclosporine can cause gingival overgrowth	• Reinforce meticulous oral hygiene • Regular scaling and recalls • Consider gingivectomy (recurrence possible)

Category	Considerations	Recommendations
3. **Pain Medication Cautions**	Opioids (e.g., Codeine, hydrocodone, oxycodone) may interact with antidiarrheals and worsen GI issues	• Avoid opioids where possible • Prefer Acetaminophen
4. **Bleeding Risk from Supplements**	Omega-3 fatty acids may increase bleeding tendency	• Exercise caution during extractions/invasive procedures • Review supplement history
5. **Metronidazole Use**	Metronidazole causes metallic taste and reacts with alcohol	• Avoid alcohol-containing mouth rinses • Advise strict alcohol avoidance during therapy
6. **Antibiotic Interactions**	Mixing bacteriostatic and bactericidal antibiotics may reduce efficacy	• If on tetracycline/ clarithromycin → prescribe clindamycin • If on metronidazole → prescribe penicillin • Do not increase existing antibiotic dose
7. **Anti-TNF Therapy – Oral Risks**	Anti-TNF biologics increase risk of opportunistic infections and lesions	• Monitor for candidiasis, ulcers, suspicious lesions (tongue, gingiva, palate) • Investigate if persistent (biopsy, sputum, immunologic tests) • Manage oral TB similar to Pulmonary Tuberculosis

4. Ulcerative Colitis

Table 1-4: Oral Manifestations in Ulcerative Colitis

Category	Condition/ Feature	Clinical Presentation	Notes
Soft Tissue Changes	Gingival & Buccal Mucosa	Swollen/oedematous mucosa	Common inflammatory finding
Ulcerative Lesions	Aphthous Ulcers	Painful oral ulcers	Seen in up to 10%; resolve during remission
Opportunistic Infections	Oral Candidiasis (Thrush)	White patches, burning sensation	Seen in severe flares or immunosuppression
Nutritional Deficiency	Vitamin B12 Deficiency	Glossitis, erythematous mucositis, pale mucosa, candidiasis	Due to malabsorption
Bleeding Risk	Coagulation Abnormality	Increased bleeding tendency	Check CBC & LFT before dental procedures

Table 1-5: Drug interactions

Drug Combination	Risk	Mechanism/ Concern	Recommendation
Mesalamine + Ibuprofen/Naproxen	Increased renal toxicity	Additive nephrotoxic effect	Avoid combination
Alternative Option – Paracetamol	—	Safer analgesic choice	Avoid Ibuprofen

5. Pseudomembranous Colitis

Table 1-6: Antibiotic Prescription Caution

Guideline	Details	Clinical Rationale
Avoid broad-spectrum antibiotics	Use only when absolutely necessary	Increases risk of Clostridioides difficile infection overgrowth
Prefer narrow-spectrum agents	e.g., Penicillin V	Lower disruption of normal gut flora
Avoid high-risk antibiotics	Especially Clindamycin, also caution with Amoxicillin	Strong association with antibiotic-associated diarrhoea
Past history consideration	History of Pseudomembranous colitis	Consult physician before prescribing

Table 1-7: Alternative Management

Approach	Details	Clinical Benefit
Non-antibiotic care	Local debridement, antiseptic rinses	Reduces need for systemic antibiotics
Referral when needed	For systemic or complex infections	Ensures safe, multidisciplinary care

Table 1-8: Probiotic Support

Recommendation	Details	Notes
Probiotics/Yogurt	Twice daily during antibiotic therapy	Helps restore gut flora balance
Timing	Give at least 2 hours apart from antibiotics	Prevents antibiotic inactivation of probiotics

Table 1-9: Patient Monitoring

Instruction	**Details**	**Clinical Importance**
Watch for diarrhoea	During or after antibiotic use	Early detection of Clostridioides difficile infection
Delayed onset awareness	Symptoms may occur days to months later	Critical for patient education
Avoid antidiarrheals	Do not use OTC anti-diarrheal drugs	Prevents toxin retention

Table 1-10: Emergency Protocol

Situation	**Action**	**Reason**
Onset of diarrhoea during antibiotics	Stop antibiotic immediately	Prevent worsening of infection
Next step	Seek urgent medical care	Early management of potential Clostridioides difficile infection

Always coordinate care with the patient's gastroenterologist or physician.

Ensure proper medical history review before procedure.

Additional Guidelines for Gastrointestinal Diseases

1. Upper GI bleeding presents as black, tarry stools (melena).
    - The Guaiac (faecal occult blood) test will be positive, indicating the presence of blood in the stool.
2. Lower GI bleeding results in the passage of fresh (bright red) blood in the stools (haematochezia).

3. Dental treatment should be avoided during an acute intestinal flare-up (e.g., inflammatory bowel disease).
    - Routine dental procedures should be deferred for 4–6 weeks following resolution of the acute episode.
4. Codeine should not be prescribed in:
    - Patients with a history of chronic constipation
    - Patients with diverticulitis
    - If narcotic analgesics are unavoidable, advise concurrent use of stool softeners.
5. In patients receiving immunosuppressive therapy:
    - Always obtain a Complete Blood Count (CBC) with:
        - Platelet count
        - White blood cell (WBC) differential
        - Calculate the Absolute Neutrophil Count (ANC) before dental treatment.
        - Follow ANC-based dental management guidelines where indicated.

ANC-Based Dental Treatment Guidelines:

ANC guidelines are especially important in patients:

- On chemotherapy
- On immunosuppressive drugs
- With leukaemia, HIV, or bone marrow disorders

Always check platelet count alongside ANC before invasive procedures.

Physician consultation is mandatory when ANC < 1000 cells/mm^3.

Table 1-11: Dental Management Based on ANC (Absolute Neutrophil Count)

ANC (cells/ mm^3)	**Dental Treatment**	**Antibiotics**	**Risk Level**	**Key Clinical Notes**
≥ 2000	All routine & invasive procedures safe	Not required	Normal	Standard precautions sufficient
1000–2000	Routine care safe; invasive procedures with caution	Consider prophylaxis (especially surgery, perio, multiple extractions)	Mild–Moderate	Assess systemic condition; use clinical judgment
< 1000	Elective care contraindicated	Required for emergency care	High	Treat only if necessary; physician consultation mandatory
< 500	No dental treatment	Required (hospital-based if emergency)	Very High	Medical stabilization first; treat only life-threatening infections

References

Anand, P.S., Nandakumar, K., & Shenoy, K.T. (2006) Are dental plaque, poor oral hygiene, and periodontal disease associated with Helicobacter pylori infection? *Journal of Periodontology*, 77, 692–698.

Ganda, K. (2013) *Dentist's Guide to Medical Conditions and Complications*, 2nd ed. Wiley-Blackwell, IA.

Gibson, N. & Ferguson, J.W. (2004) Steroid cover for dental patients on long-term steroid medication: proposed clinical guidelines based upon a critical review of the literature. *British Dental Journal*, 197, 681–685.

Khalaf, M.W., Khader, R., Cobetto, G. *et al.* (2013) Risk of adrenal crisis in dental patients. *Results of a systematic search of the literature. Journal of the American Dental Association*, 144, 152–160.

Kilmartin, C.M. (2002) Dental implications of Helicobacter pylori. *Journal of the Canadian Dental Association*, 68, 489–493.

Malahias, T., Cheng, J., Brar, P. *et al.* (2009) The association between celiac disease, dental enamel defects and aphthous ulcers in a United States cohort. *Journal of Clinical Gastroenterology*, 44, 191–194.

McGrath, E., Bardsley, P., & Basran, G. (2008) Black hairy tongue: what is your call? *Journal Canadian Medical Association MAJ*, 178, 1137–1138.

Miller, C.S., Little, J.W., & Falace, D.A. (2001) Supplemental corticosteroids for dental patients with adrenal insufficiency. Reconsideration of the problem. *Journal of the American Dental Association*, 132, 1570–1570.

Nasrolahel, M., Maleki, I., & Emadian, O. (2003) *Helicobacter pylori* colonization in dental plaque and gastric infection. *Romanian Journal of Gastroenterology*, 12, 293–299.

Pontes, H.A., Neto, N.C., Ferreira, K.B. *et al.* (2009) Oral manifestations of vitamin B12 deficiency: a case report. *Journal of the Canadian Dental Association*, 75, 533–537.

Chapter 2

Dental Management of Patients with Respiratory Disorders

Introduction

Respiratory disorders can significantly influence dental care, requiring modifications in treatment approach and patient management. Conditions like Chronic Obstructive Pulmonary Disease and Asthma often necessitate treating patients in an upright position due to breathing difficulty and may increase the risk of pulmonary infections from oral pathogens, especially in the presence of poor periodontal health. Asthma medications, particularly inhaled β-agonists, can lead to oral issues such as xerostomia, candidiasis, caries, and gingivitis. Although oral manifestations of Tuberculosis are rare, they can mimic serious conditions like carcinoma, making accurate diagnosis essential. Dentists also play a role in managing Obstructive Sleep Apnoea Syndrome through oral appliances that advance the mandible.

Dental Management of Patients with Respiratory Disorders

1. Asthma

Table 2-1-1: Interactions of Asthma medications with antibiotics

Antibiotic	Asthma Medication(s)	Interaction/Risk	Management Recommendation
Erythromycin	Theophylline	↓ CYP metabolism → ↑ theophylline levels → toxicity	Avoid combination; choose alternative antibiotic
Erythromycin	Albuterol	↑ risk QT prolongation & arrhythmias (via hypokalaemia)	If used, monitor ECG & electrolytes; preferably use different antibiotic
Erythromycin	Inhaled levalbuterol or pirbuterol	↑ risk QT prolongation & arrhythmias	Monitor therapy closely or switch antibiotic
Erythromycin	Zafirlukast, zileuton, montelukast	↓ hepatic metabolism → ↑ leukotriene-modifier levels	Use with caution; consider alternate antibiotic
Erythromycin	Systemic corticosteroids	↑ risk QT prolongation & arrhythmias (via hypokalemia)	Monitor or select a different antibiotic
Azole antifungals (Fluconazole)	Theophylline	↓ CYP metabolism → ↑ theophylline levels → toxicity	Monitor theophylline serum levels; adjust dose in consultation
Azithromycin	Mometasone/ Formoterol	↑ risk QT prolongation & arrhythmias; possible steroid potentiation	Avoid if possible; monitor potassium & cardiac status

(Contd.)

Antibiotic	Asthma Medication(s)	Interaction/Risk	Management Recommendation
Azithromycin	Inhaled levalbuterol or pirbuterol	↑ risk QT prolongation & arrhythmias	Monitor or choose another antibiotic
Azithromycin	Systemic corticosteroids	↑ risk QT prolongation & arrhythmias	Monitor or choose another antibiotic
Clarithromycin	Mometasone/ formoterol	↑ steroid levels → Cushing syndrome/adrenal suppression; ↑ arrhythmias	Avoid; use alternative antibiotic
Clarithromycin	Inhaled levalbuterol or pirbuterol	↑ risk QT prolongation & arrhythmias	Monitor or choose another antibiotic
Clarithromycin	Systemic corticosteroids	↑ risk QT prolongation & arrhythmias	Monitor or choose another antibiotic

Key Points

- QT Prolongation & Arrhythmias

  Macrolides (erythro-, azithro-, clarithro-) can inhibit cardiac potassium channels and potentiate hypokalaemia (especially when given with β2-agonists or steroids). Always assess cardiac history and consider baseline/periodic ECG and serum electrolytes if co-administration is unavoidable.

- Theophylline Toxicity

  Any strong CYP1A2 inhibitor (erythromycin, fluconazole, etc.) can markedly increase theophylline levels, risking nausea, seizures, or arrhythmias. If theophylline use is essential, coordinate with the patient's physician to monitor serum levels and adjust dosing.

- Steroid Potentiation

  Clarithromycin can inhibit metabolism of systemically absorbed corticosteroids, elevating systemic steroid exposure. When systemic steroids are used, choose an antibiotic without CYP3A4 inhibition (Azithromycin/Metronidazole).

- Practical Tips

  1. Review patient's full medication list before prescribing antibiotics.
  2. Prefer antibiotics with minimal CYP interactions (e.g., penicillins, cephalosporins) when possible.
  3. Communicate with the patient's physician if potentially interacting drugs are unavoidable—consider lab monitoring or dose adjustments.
  4. Document any interaction concerns and the plan (e.g., "prescribed cephalexin instead of erythromycin due to theophylline use

Table 2-1-2: Interactions of Asthma medications with: Aspirin, NSAIDs and Narcotics

Aspect	Details	Clinical Notes
Condition	Aspirin-Exacerbated Respiratory Disease (AERD)	Affects ~3–5% of asthma patients
Key Features	Chronic eosinophilic sinusitis, nasal polyposis, asthma, sensitivity to COX-1 inhibitors	Classic tetrad of AERD
Triggering Drugs	Aspirin, NSAIDs	COX-1 inhibition mechanism
Clinical Presentation	Bronchoconstriction, nasal congestion within 30 min–3 hrs	Acute hypersensitivity reaction
Management	Avoid aspirin & traditional NSAIDs	Use only if tolerance proven or under specialist care
Drug Example	Codeine	Less preferred dental analgesic

(Contd.)

Aspect	Details	Clinical Notes
Risk	Respiratory depression	Can worsen asthma
Clinical Concern	May precipitate asthma exacerbation	Especially during active episode
Recommendation	Avoid in unstable asthma or acute attacks	Prefer non-opioid alternatives

Table 2-1-3: Interactions of Asthma medications with Epinephrine in Local anaesthetic

Aspect	Details	Clinical Notes
Use in Dentistry	Present in local anaesthetics as vasoconstrictor	Improves duration & reduces bleeding
Additive Concern	Sodium metabisulphite (preservative)	Can trigger reactions in sulphite-sensitive asthma patients
Drug	Epinephrine	Sympathomimetic agent
Pharmacologic Action	Beta-2 receptor stimulation → bronchodilation	Beneficial in asthma
Emergency Use	1:1000 concentration, 0.5–1.0 mL IM	First-line in acute severe asthma/anaphylaxis

Summary of Clinical Recommendations

- Avoid aspirin and NSAIDs in asthmatics unless tolerance is confirmed.
- Do not use codeine during or shortly after an asthma attack.
- Be cautious with epinephrine-containing anaesthetics in sulphite-sensitive asthmatics.
- Recognize epinephrine's bronchodilatory role in emergency asthma management.

Dental Notes: Management of the Asthmatic Patient

Table 2-1-3: Recommendation in Asthma Patients

Aspect	Recommendation
Medical History	• Take thorough history at each visit.
	• Document the last attack and its trigger.
	• Postpone dental treatment if increased emergency visits or poor asthma control.
Asthma Severity	• Assess asthma severity before treatment.
	• Postpone elective treatment if symptomatic (wheezing/coughing).
Inhalers & Emergency Kit	• Ensure the patient's inhaler is within reach during treatment.
	• Use emergency kit inhaler if the patient forgot theirs.
	• Keep oxygen and a bronchodilator in the emergency kit.
Medications	• Corticosteroids: Monitor for infections and diabetes risk.
	• Nitrous Oxide: Consider for mild to moderate asthma; consult physician before use.
	• Bronchodilators: Ensure availability and monitor.
Dental Treatment Considerations	• Avoid triggers (sealants, aerosol irritants, methyl methacrylate, etc.).
	• Use rubber dam to reduce irritants.
	• Avoid prolonged supine position during treatment.
	• Use local anaesthetics with epinephrine cautiously.
Xerostomia	• Monitor for dry mouth due to inhalers and medications.
	• Encourage water intake, fluoride use, and salivary substitutes.

(Contd.)

Aspect	**Recommendation**
Oral Hygiene	• Reinforce daily oral hygiene to prevent gingivitis.
	• Instruct patient to rinse and brush teeth after inhaler use to avoid oral candidiasis.
Pain Management	• Avoid NSAIDs and aspirin due to the risk of triggering asthma.
	• Use acetaminophen as the analgesic of choice.
Preventive Measures	• Regularly review asthma management plan and ensure emergency procedures and medication are in place.

2. Chronic Obstructive Pulmonary Disease (COPD)

Table 2-2: Consideration and Management of COPD Patient

Area of Focus	**Management/Consideration**
Drug Interactions	Azithromycin + formoterol can increase QT prolongation and arrhythmias. Monitor or use alternative antibiotics.
Medications & Drug Precautions	Avoid narcotics and barbiturates (cause respiratory depression). Always ask about current medications at each visit.
Breathing Assessment	Monitor breathing pattern. Postpone elective dental treatment if symptoms like breathlessness, productive cough, or cyanosis are present.
Positioning	Avoid supine position if uncomfortable. Opt for upright or semi-supine positioning to avoid orthopnea. Ensure space for oxygen tanks if necessary.
Use of Local Anaesthetics	No contraindications for therapeutic doses in COPD patients.
Comorbidities	COPD patients with emphysema may have comorbidities like hypertension or heart failure.
General Anaesthesia	Use with caution in moderate to severe COPD due to respiratory depression. Consult physician before use.

Area of Focus	Management/Consideration
Use of Nitrous Oxide	Safe for mild to moderate emphysema with low oxygen; avoid in severe cases. Consult with physician.
Xerostomia & Oral Health	COPD medications (e.g., anticholinergics) can cause dry mouth. Encourage increased water intake, salivary substitutes, and fluoride application.
Oral Candidiasis Prevention	Patients using inhaled corticosteroids should rinse and brush teeth after each use to prevent oral fungal infections.

3. Tuberculosis (TB)

Table 2-3-1: Management in TB Patient

Category	Details
Drug-Drug Interactions	
Acetaminophen + Isoniazid	Increased risk of hepatotoxicity. Caution advised but not contraindicated.
Clarithromycin/ Erythromycin + Isoniazid	May increase clarithromycin levels and risk of QT prolongation/arrhythmias. Best to use azithromycin if macrolide is needed.
Epinephrine + Isoniazid	No known interactions.

Table 2-3-2: Dental Management in TB Patient

Category	Considerations	Recommendations
1. Medical History	Identify risk factors (e.g., HIV, IV drug use, crowded living/working conditions)	Take detailed history; assess TB risk before treatment
2. Past TB Infection/ Treatment	Previous TB or incomplete treatment history	Document clearly; evaluate current disease status
3. Health Authority Clearance	Active TB cases are notifiable diseases	Obtain clearance/letter from public health authority before elective care

(Contd.)

Category	Considerations	Recommendations
4. Drug Therapy – Isoniazid	Isoniazid may cause hepatotoxicity	Consult physician; monitor liver function tests (monthly recommended)
5. Active TB	Patient is infectious	**Defer all elective dental treatment**; physician consultation mandatory
6. Emergency Treatment	Urgent care may be required in infectious patients	Treat in hospital setting with airborne infection isolation Use N95 respirators and strict infection control
7. Treated/ Asymptomatic TB	Positive PPD + completed therapy + negative follow-up chest X-ray	Routine dental care can be provided with standard precautions
8. Infection Control	Risk of airborne transmission	Follow strict standard precautions Minimize aerosol-generating procedures where possible
9. History of Active TB	Previously treated TB cases	Medical consult before dental treatment to confirm non-infectious status
10. Associated Systemic Consideration	Link between Obstructive Sleep Apnea and Nonarteritic Anterior Ischemic Optic Neuropathy	Consider referral to ophthalmologist if visual symptoms or risk factors present

4. Obstructive Sleep Apnoea

Table 2-4: Dental Consideration in Sleep Apnoea Patients

Section	Details
Clinical Synopsis	OSA is characterized by repeated episodes of airway obstruction lasting >10 seconds, causing gaps in breathing. Common in both children and adults.

Section	Details
Risk Factors	Obesity- Hypertension- Habitual snoring- Daytime hypersomnolence- Adenotonsillar hypertrophy in children
Risk Indicators in Primary Care	Patients with two of the following: - Snoring- Persistent daytime sleepiness/drowsiness (e.g., while driving)- Obesity or hypertension. Also consider diabetes or GERD.
Medications Prescribed	No medications for OSA treatment. Treatment options include: 1. CPAP therapy2. Surgery (for severe cases)3. Positional therapy4. Alcohol avoidance5. Weight loss
Oral Appliances	AASM recommends oral appliances for mild to moderate OSA, including: - Mandibular advancement appliances (moves mandible forward)- Tongue-retaining devices (moves tongue forward)
Dental Notes	1. Perform intra- and extraoral examination to check for OSA indicators. 2. Oral appliances are within the scope of dentistry. 3. Watch for xerostomia, TMJ, bruxism, and periodontal issues.
Common OSA-Related Dental Issues	Xerostomia (dry mouth)- TMJ problems- Periodontal issues- Bruxism (teeth grinding)- Narrow palates and anterior tooth crowding (mainly in children)
Sleepiness in Dental Settings	Patients with OSA may fall asleep in the dental chair or waiting room due to excessive daytime sleepiness.
Positioning in Dental Chair	Avoid the supine position to reduce airway obstruction risk.
Sleep Study Requirement	A physician's sleep study may be required for diagnosis before dental treatment.
Active Screening by Dentists	Dentists should actively screen for OSA in patients.
Snore Appliance Caution	Never make a snore appliance without a prior sleep apnoea test.

References

Araujo, M.W. & Andreana, S. (2002) Risk and prevention of transmission of infectious diseases in dentistry. *Quintessence International*, 33, 376–382.

Bencome, J. & Castellanos, S. (2011) Sleep apnea syndrome. *Registered Dental Hygienist*, 31, 76–77, 115.

Budenz, A.W. (2008) Local anesthetics and medically compromised patients. *Journal of the California Dental Association*, 28, 611–619.

Coke, J.M. & Karaki, D.T. (2002) The asthma patient and dental management. *General Dentistry*, 50, 504–507.

Diaz-Guzman, L.M. (2001) Management of the dental patient with pulmonary tuberculosis. *Medicina Oral*, 6, 124–134.

Dort, L.C. (2003) When patients fall asleep in the dental chair—a wake-up call for dentists. *Journal of the Canadian Dental Association*, 69, 14–15.

Harrel, S.K. (2003) Contaminated dental aerosols: the risks and implications for dental hygienists. *Dimensions of Dental Hygiene*, 1 (6), 16–20.

Harrel, S.K. & Molinari, J. (2004) Aerosols and splatter in dentistry: a brief review of the literature and infection control implications. *The Journal of the American Dental Association*, 135, 429–437.

Hupp, W.S. (2006) Dental management of patients with obstructive pulmonary disease. *Dental Clinics of North America*, 50, 513–527.

Khalaf, M.W., Khader, R., Cobetto, G. *et al.* (2013) Risk of adrenal crisis in dental patients. *Journal of the American Dental Association*, 144 (2), 152–160.

Kratt, M. (2010) The relationship between sleep apnea and dentistry. *Dentistry IQ Network*. http://www.dentistryiq.com/articles/2010/06/the-relationship-between.html [accessed April 10, 2013].

Lozano, A.C., Sarrion Perez, M.G., & Esteve, C.G. (2011): Dental considerations in patients with respiratory problems. *Journal Clinical Experimental Dentistry*, 3 (3), e222–e227.

Padma, A., Ramakrishnan, N., & Narayanan, V. (2007) Management of obstructive sleep apnea: a dental perspective. *Indian Journal of Dental Research* 18, 201–209.

Perusse, R., Goulet, J.P., & Turcotte, J.-Y. (1992) Contraindications to vasoconstrictors in dentistry: Part II. *Oral Surgery Oral Medicine Oral Pathology*, 74, 687–691.

Robbins, M.L. (2009) Tuberculosis in your dental practice: can it happen? *Journal of the Tennessee Dental Association*, 89, 22–25.

Steinbacher, D.M. & Glick, M. (2001) The dental patient with asthma. *An update and oral health consideration. Journal of the American Dental Association*, 132 (9), 1229–1239.

Chapter 3

Dental Management of Patients with Renal Disorders

Introduction

Dental management for patients with renal disorders is complex and requires close collaboration between the dentist and the patient's nephrologist to address risks of bleeding, infection, and altered drug metabolism. Key considerations include timing procedures around dialysis schedules and adjusting medications that the kidneys would normally filter.

Dental Management of Patients with Renal Disorders

Acute renal injury (AKI) is a sudden decline in kidney function, usually due to causes like dehydration, shock, or trauma, leading to reduced urine output and a rapid rise in serum creatinine, and is often reversible if treated early. In contrast, chronic kidney disease (CKD) is a progressive, irreversible loss of kidney function lasting ≥3 months, most commonly caused by diabetes and hypertension, and may eventually progress to end-stage renal disease (ESRD) requiring dialysis or transplantation. Kidney function is assessed primarily by glomerular filtration rate (GFR), with decreased GFR and increased creatinine and blood urea nitrogen indicating impairment. CKD leads to multiple complications such as uraemia, anaemia, immune suppression, and bone disorders due to impaired vitamin D activation and secondary hyperparathyroidism. Patients often present with oral manifestations like xerostomia, halitosis, and mucosal changes. Management includes controlling underlying diseases and using medications like antihypertensives, diuretics, erythropoietin, statins, and vitamin D, with careful monitoring and dose adjustment based on kidney function.

Chronic Kidney Disease

Table 3-1: Dental management in Chronic kidney disease

Aspect	Key Points	Dental Considerations
General Considerations	CKD causes bleeding tendency, anaemia, hypertension, infection risk, altered drug metabolism	Obtain CBC, Hb, Hematocrit (Hct), WBC, platelets, ferritin, reticulocyte count
Drug Prescribing	Altered pharmacokinetics (absorption, metabolism, excretion)	Assess GFR before prescribing; adjust dose & interval
	NSAIDs	Avoid long-term use
	Codeine	Avoid in renal failure/dialysis
	Lidocaine	Safe
	Carbocaine (Mepivacaine)	Risk of toxicity (renal excretion)
Bleeding Risk	Due to anaemia, thrombocytopenia, platelet dysfunction, uraemia	Check platelet count & haematocrit (≥30%)
		Expect bleeding during procedures
		Use local haemostatic measures
		Severe cases → platelet transfusion/Desmopressin (DDAVP)
		Delay elective procedures if abnormal

(Contd.)

Aspect	Key Points	Dental Considerations
Anaemia	Normocytic anaemia (GFR <60 mL/min) due to ↓ erythropoietin	Check Hb/Hct before invasive procedures
	Treatment	Erythropoietin (epoetin alfa), darbepoetin, iron supplements
	Drug Interaction	Iron + tetracycline/ doxycycline → separate by ≥ 2 hrs
Infection Risk	Leukopenia → increased susceptibility	Monitor oral infections; consider antibiotic prophylaxis (consult physician)
Hypertension	Common in CKD (cause & effect)	Monitor BP before & after procedures
	Medications	Diuretics, ACE inhibitors, ARBs
	Oral Effects	Xerostomia, orthostatic hypotension
		Make the patient sit upright before discharge
Diabetes (Comorbidity)	Common in CKD	Patients may be on insulin/ oral hypoglycaemics
		Watch for neuropathy & delayed healing
Periodontal Disease	Chronic inflammation link with CKD/ESRD	Increased plaque, calculus, gingival inflammation
		Treat periodontal disease actively
Dental Caries	Increased incidence	Regular monitoring; fluoride supplementation
Vitamin D Deficiency	Common in CKD; linked to periodontal disease	Monitor and manage deficiency

Kidney Dialysis

Table 3-2: Purpose of Kidney Dialysis medications

Medication	Purpose/Indication
Erythropoietin (EPO)	Treats anaemia by stimulating red blood cell production
Iron Supplements	Supports erythropoietin function and treats iron deficiency anaemia
Phosphate Binders (e.g., Calcium Carbonate)	Maintains serum phosphate levels and prevents phosphate build-up
Water-Soluble Vitamins (e.g., Vitamin C, B-complex, Folic Acid)	Replaces vitamins lost during dialysis
HMG-CoA Reductase Inhibitors (Statins)	Manages cholesterol levels and reduces cardiovascular risk
Antidiabetic Medications (Oral or Insulin)	Controls blood sugar levels in dialysis patients with diabetes

Table 3-3: Dental Considerations in Kidney Dialysis Patients

Consideration	Details
1. Nephrologist Consult	Obtain a consult to assess the patient's kidney function status.
2. Major Considerations	Focus on bleeding, infection, and medication use.
3. Antibiotic Prophylaxis	AHA guidelines suggest prophylaxis due to the risk of dental infections and infective endocarditis.
4. Lab Values	Obtain current CBC to evaluate bleeding risk.
5. Uremic Bleeding	Occurs if dialysis is inadequate; many patients will have dialysis before dental visits, reducing risk.
6. Medication Dosing	Adjust medications based on the patient's current GFR.
7. Dialyzable Antibiotics	Antibiotics like amoxicillin, amoxicillin/clavulanate, and metronidazole can be taken after dialysis.
8. Periodontal Health	Monitor and manage periodontal conditions in haemodialysis patients.

(Contd.)

Consideration	Details
9. Infection Risks	Increased risk for candidiasis and herpes infections due to immunosuppression.
10. Hepatitis Risk	Higher incidence of hepatitis B and C among dialysis patients.
11. Timing of Dental Appointments	Schedule dental appointments 24 hours after haemodialysis to allow heparin clearance. (Preferably morning time)
12. AV Fistula Consideration	Do not measure blood pressure on the arm with the AV fistula.

Kidney Transplant

Table 3-4: Medications for Kidney Transplant Patients – Dental Considerations

Medication	Mechanism/ Purpose	Adverse Effects/ Warnings	Dental Implications
Azathioprine	Antimetabolite; inhibits rapidly dividing cells to prevent graft rejection	• Bone marrow suppression • Increased infection risk • Malignancy risk	• Obtain recent CBC before invasive procedures • Monitor for bleeding, oral ulcers, infections • Strict asepsis • Medical consult recommended
Tacrolimus	Calcineurin inhibitor; suppresses T-cell activation	• Increased infection risk • Lymphoma risk • Hypertension • Nephrotoxicity	• Monitor for opportunistic oral infections (candidiasis, herpes) • Gingival enlargement possible (↑ if combined with CCBs) • Physician consult for invasive care

Medication	Mechanism/ Purpose	Adverse Effects/ Warnings	Dental Implications
Cyclosporine	Calcineurin inhibitor; suppresses T-cell function and prolongs graft survival	• Nephrotoxicity • Hepatotoxicity • Hypertension • Gingival overgrowth	• Gingival enlargement common (especially with Nifedipine) • Emphasize meticulous oral hygiene • Frequent recalls (≈3 months) • Consider gingivectomy if severe

Table 3-5: Interactions of Dental Drugs with Kidney Transplant Drugs

Dental Drug	Kidney Transplant Drug	Interaction/Risk	Management/ Recommendation
Clarithromycin/ Erythromycin	Cyclosporine, Tacrolimus	↑ Immunosuppressant levels → toxicity, QT prolongation	AVOID—use Azithromycin or Clindamycin instead
Ciprofloxacin (Cipro)	Cyclosporine	↑ Cyclosporine levels → nephrotoxicity	AVOID
Clindamycin	Mycophenolate	May ↓ mycophenolate levels	Use with caution, monitor efficacy
Azole Antifungals (e.g., fluconazole, ketoconazole)	Cyclosporine, Tacrolimus, Sirolimus	↑ Immunosuppressant levels → nephrotoxicity, neurotoxicity	Consult nephrologist, may need dose adjustment
Azole Antifungals	Statins (CYP3A4 substrates)	↑ Statin levels → myopathy, rhabdomyolysis	AVOID
Azole Antifungals + Systemic Corticosteroids	Cyclosporine, Tacrolimus, Sirolimus	↑ Risk of adrenal insufficiency	Consult nephrologist

(Contd.)

Dental Drug	Kidney Transplant Drug	Interaction/Risk	Management/ Recommendation
Metronidazole	Mycophenolate	May ↑ mycophenolate levels	Use with caution, monitor for toxicity
Tetracycline	Mycophenolate	May ↓ mycophenolate levels	Use with caution, monitor efficacy
Azithromycin/ Clarithromycin/ Erythromycin	Mycophenolate	May ↓ mycophenolate levels	Use with caution, monitor efficacy
Acyclovir/ Valacyclovir	Mycophenolate	↑ Levels of both → toxicity	Monitor kidney function, adjust if needed
Systemic Corticosteroids	Mycophenolate	↑ Risk of immunosuppression → infection	Use cautiously

Table 3-6: Dental Management Chart: Patients with Kidney Disease

Category	Key Considerations
Medical Coordination	• Mandatory consult with nephrologist • Continuous communication with transplant team
Assessment Questions	• GFR/Creatinine clearance (CrCl) • Current medications (e.g., Cyclosporine, Tacrolimus, Azathioprine) • Platelet count - Dialysis status - Transplant list status
Blood Pressure	• Monitor and control hypertension (common in renal patients)
Bleeding Risk	• Uraemia → decreased platelet function • Check CBC & coagulation profile • Platelet transfusion may be required for major procedures
Scheduling Care	• Best scheduled **day after dialysis** (reduced bleeding, toxin levels lower)

Category	Key Considerations
Local Anaesthetics	• Generally safe (no dose adjustment needed) • Amide & ester anaesthetics metabolized outside kidneys
Analgesics	• Acetaminophen = safest choice • Avoid NSAIDs/aspirin unless approved • Fentanyl preferred if strong analgesia needed • Avoid Codeine if GFR <50 or ESRD
Antibiotics	• Prophylaxis often needed (immunosuppressed) • Safe: Azithromycin, Clindamycin, Doxycycline, Pen VK • Avoid tetracycline (accumulates in renal impairment)
Oral Infections	• Must be eliminated before transplant (source of systemic infection)
Gingival Overgrowth	• Common with Cyclosporine and calcium channel blockers • Manage with strict oral hygiene, scaling, possible gingivectomy
Drug Interactions	• Check interactions with immunosuppressants (cyclosporine, tacrolimus, azathioprine, corticosteroids, mycophenolate)
Oral Hygiene	• Critical for both transplant candidates and recipients • Frequent recalls (every 3 months recommended)

Table 3-7: Dose adjustments of dental drugs in renal diseases

Drug	GFR >50 ml/min	GFR 10–50 ml/min	GFR <10 ml/min (ESRD)
Antibiotics			
Amoxicillin	250–500 mg q8h	250–500 mg q8–12h	q24h
Amoxicillin/ Clavulanate	250–500 mg q8h; 875 mg q12h	250–500 mg q12h	q24h
Azithromycin	500 mg daily	No adjustment	Use with caution
Clarithromycin	250–500 mg q12h	↓ dose 50%	↓ dose 50%

(Contd.)

Drug	**GFR >50 ml/min**	**GFR 10–50 ml/min**	**GFR <10 ml/min (ESRD)**
Ciprofloxacin	500–700 mg q12h	↓ 50–75%	↓ 50%
Clindamycin	300 mg TID	No adjustment	No adjustment
Metronidazole	500 mg q8h	No adjustment	No adjustment
Doxycycline	100 mg BID	No adjustment	No adjustment
Tetracycline	250 mg q6–8h	q12–24h	Avoid
Penicillin VK	250–500 mg q6h	No adjustment	No adjustment
Antivirals			
Acyclovir (oral)	200–800 mg q4–12h	No adjustment	200 mg q12h
Valacyclovir	500 mg q12h	500 mg q12–24h	500 mg q24h
Antifungals			
Fluconazole	200–400 mg q24h	↓ dose 50%	↓ dose 50%
Analgesics			
Acetaminophen	500 mg q4h	q6h	q8h
Aspirin	q4–6h	q4–6h	Avoid
Ibuprofen	↓ 50–75%; avoid	Caution long-term	Avoid
Naproxen	↓ 50–75%; avoid	Avoid	Avoid
Diflunisal	No change	↓ dose 50%	↓ dose 50%
Codeine/ Acetaminophen	30–60 mg q4–6h	Consider ↓ dose or avoid	Avoid
Hydrocodone/ Acetaminophen	50–100% dose	↓ 50–75%; caution	↓ 25%; caution
Oxycodone/ Acetaminophen	No change	↓ 50–75%; caution	Avoid
Fentanyl	100% dose	↓ 25%	Avoid
Tramadol	Normal dose	IR: 50–100 mg q12h or avoid; ER: Avoid	Avoid

Drug	**GFR >50 ml/min**	**GFR 10–50 ml/min**	**GFR <10 ml/min (ESRD)**
Local Anaesthetics			
Lidocaine	No adjustment	No adjustment	No adjustment
Mepivacaine (Carbocaine)	No adjustment	Caution with repeated doses	Caution—limited data
Articaine (Septocaine)	No precautions (except hypoxia)	No precautions (except hypoxia)	No precautions (except hypoxia)
Oral Sedatives			
Diazepam	No change	Start low; caution in chronic use	Start low; titrate cautiously
Midazolam	0.5–2 mg IV over 2 min; titrate	No adjustment; caution	Use with caution

References

Álamo, S.A., Esteve, C.G., & Pérez, M.G.S. (2011) Dental considerations for the patient with renal disease. *Journal of Clinical Experimental Dentistry*, 3, e112–e119.

Al-Badr, W. & Martin, K.J. (2008) Vitamin D and kidney disease. *Clinical Journal of the American Society of Nephrology*, 3, 1555–1560.

Brockmann, W. & Badr, M. (2010) Chronic kidney disease. Pharmacological considerations for the dentist. *The Journal of the American Dental Association*, 141 (11), 1330–1339.

Buckley, D.J., Barrett, A.P., Koutta, J. *et al.* (1986) Control of bleeding in severely uremic patients undergoing oral surgery. *Oral Surgery Oral Medicine Oral Pathology*, 61, 546–549.

Caster, D.J., Loughran, J.H., & Kinane, D.F. (2010) Dental and medical comanagement of osteoporosis, kidney disease, and cancer. In: R.J. Genco & R.C. Williams (eds), 1st ed, Chapter 17, pp. 270–287. *Periodontal Diseases and Overall Health: A Clinician's Guide.* Professional Audience Communications, Inc., Yardley, PA.

Cervero, A.J., Bagan, J.V., Sorian, J.Y. *et al.* (2008) Dental management in renal failure: patients on dialysis. *Medicina Oral Patologia Oral y Cirugia Bucal*, 13 (7), E419–E426.

Cox, B., Durieux, M.E., & Marcus, M.A.E. (2003) Toxicity of local anesthetics. *Best Practice & Research Clinical Anaesthesiology*, 17, 111–136.

Craig, R. (2008) Interactions between chronic renal disease and periodontal disease. *Oral Diseases*, 14, 1–7.

De Rossi, S.S. & Glick, M. (1996) Dental considerations for the patient with renal disease receiving hemodialysis. *Journal of the American Dental Association*, 127, 211–219.

De Souza, C.M., Braosi, A.P.R., Luczyszyn, S.M. *et al.* (2014) Association between oral health parameters, periodontitis and its treatment and mortality in hemodialysis patients. *Journal of Periodontology*, 85(6), e169–e178.

Fletcher, P.D., Scopp, I.W., & Hersch, R.A. (1977) Oral manifestations of secondary hyperparathyroidism related to long-term haemodialysis therapy. *Journal of Oral Surgery*, 43, 218–226.

Ismail, G., Dumitriu, H.T., Dumitriu, A.S. *et al.* (2013) Periodontal disease: a convert source of inflammation in chronic kidney disease patients. *International Journal of Nephrology*, 2013, 515796.

King, E. (2013) Dental management of patients in end stage renal failure on dialysis. *Journal of the Michigan Dental Association*, 59, 42–45.

Klassen, J.T. & Karsko, B.M. (2009) The dental health status of dialysis patients. *The Journal of the Canadian Dental Association*, 68, 34–38.

Patil, S., Khaandelwal, S., Doni, B. *et al.* (2012) Oral manifestations in chronic renal failure patients attending two hospitals in North Karnataka, India. *Oral Health and Dental Management*, 11, 100–106.

Rivera, J.A., O'Hare, A. M., & Harper, G.M. (2012) Update on the management of chronic kidney disease.

Sulejmanagic, H., Sulejmanagic, N., Prohic, S. *et al.* (2005). Dental treatment of patients with kidney diseases—review. *Bosnian Journal of Basic Medical Sciences*, 5 (1), 52–56.

Tong, D.C. & Walker, R.J. (2004) Antibiotic prophylaxis in dialysis patients undergoing invasive dental procedures. *Nephrology*, 9, 167–170.

Chapter 4

Dental Management of Patients with Hepatic Disorders

Introduction

Dental management of patients with hepatic disorders requires careful assessment of coagulation status, drug metabolism, and infection risk. Clinicians must consult with a hepatologist for high-risk patients, utilize local haemostatic measures for bleeding control, and adjust drug dosages or avoid hepatotoxic medications like acetaminophen and NSAIDs.

Drug Metabolism by the Liver (Dental Perspective) – Why is it important?

- Drugs that are primarily cleared by the liver may require dose adjustment in patients with hepatic impairment.
- Clinically significant changes in drug metabolism usually occur only in advanced/severe liver disease.
- Most drugs are metabolized by hepatic cytochrome P450 (CYP450) enzymes.
  - In liver disease, the liver may be unable to synthesize adequate amounts of these microsomal enzymes, leading to altered pharmacokinetics.

Assessment of Liver Function

- Unlike renal disease (where creatinine clearance and GFR guide dosage adjustment), reliable indicators of hepatic drug-metabolizing capacity are lacking.

- Liver enzymes:
  - AST, ALT, GGT
  - ALP
- These tests indicate hepatocellular injury or cholestasis, but do NOT reflect the liver's ability to metabolize drugs.

Dosage Adjustment in Liver Disease

If dose modification is required:

- Reduce the drug dose, or
- Increase the dosing interval
- Always consult the patient's physician before making adjustments

Drug Elimination Pathways

- All drugs must be eliminated from the body:
  - Either metabolized to water-soluble compounds (mostly in the liver)
  - Or excreted unchanged
- Most drugs:
  - Metabolized in the liver
  - Excreted by the kidneys in urine

Local Anaesthetics and Liver Disease

Amide local anaesthetics metabolized in the liver:

- Lidocaine
- Mepivacaine
- Bupivacaine
- Prilocaine

Mild to moderate liver disease:

- Generally, well tolerated

Severe liver disease:

- Dosage reduction may be required

Lidocaine Guideline

- Maximum of 3 cartridges of 2% lidocaine is considered safe

Consultation with the hepatologist is recommended

Patient with Liver Disease

Medical consultation is essential to determine:

- Severity of liver impairment
- Bleeding tendency
- Need for drug dosage modification

Complete blood count (CBC) with differential, including:

- Platelet count
- White blood cell (WBC) count

Antibiotic Prophylaxis & Infection Control

- There is no strong evidence-based guideline supporting routine antibiotic prophylaxis in all patients with liver disease.
- Antibiotic prophylaxis may be considered based on:
  - Overall medical status
  - Presence of active oral infection
  - Decreased WBC count
  - Immunosuppression
- Physician consultation is recommended before prescribing antibiotics
- Patients with liver disease have an increased risk of infection, reported to be as high as 30%.

Infection Control Measures

- Strict adherence to universal precautions to prevent cross-infection
- Meticulous aseptic technique during all dental procedure.

Table 4-1: Dental Drugs Metabolized in the Liver – Clinical Guide

Category	Drug	Recommendation	Clinical Notes
Analgesics/Anti-inflammatory	Acetaminophen	Use cautiously, ≤2 g/day	Avoid chronic use
	Aspirin	Avoid	↑ Bleeding risk
	Ibuprofen	Avoid in severe liver disease	Risk in hepatitis/cirrhosis
	Naproxen	Not recommended	Hepatic risk
	Codeine (+ acetaminophen)	Reduce dose/avoid	Risk of accumulation
	Hydrocodone (+ acetaminophen)	Limit to 2–3 days	Avoid long-term use
Antibiotics	Amoxicillin	Safe	Standard dose
	Amoxicillin-clavulanate	Avoid if prior hepatic injury	Clavulanate-related toxicity
	Penicillin V	Safe	Standard dose
	Azithromycin	Avoid	Hepatic metabolism concern
	Clarithromycin	No adjustment	Generally safe
	Clindamycin	Reduce 50% in cirrhosis	No change in hepatitis
	Erythromycin	Avoid	Hepatotoxic (estolate form)
	Metronidazole	Reduce/avoid in severe disease	Safe in mild cases
	Fluconazole	No adjustment (mild–moderate)	Monitor liver
	Tetracycline	Avoid	Hepatotoxic risk
	Doxycycline	Use cautiously	Prefer alternatives

(Contd.)

Category	Drug	Recommendation	Clinical Notes
Local Anaesthetics	Lidocaine, mepivacaine, bupivacaine, prilocaine	Safe in mild–moderate disease	Reduce dose in severe disease
		Max: ~3 cartridges (2% lidocaine)	Avoid overdose
General Anaesthetics	Halothane, thiopentone	Avoid	Hepatotoxic
	Isoflurane, nitrous oxide	Acceptable	Safer options
Sedatives/ Anxiolytics	Diazepam, Midazolam, Alprazolam	Acceptable	Use lowest effective dose

Table 4-2: Platelets, Bleeding Tendency & Liver Disease – Dental Management

Category	Subcategory	Details/Guidelines	Clinical Notes
Platelet Count	< 50,000/mm^3	Significant bleeding risk	Defer invasive procedures if possible
	Management	Consider platelet transfusion to raise >50,000/mm^3	Commonly recommended
Platelet Transfusion	Timing	Immediate rise in platelet count	Peak at ~1 hour
	Dental Scheduling	Perform procedure soon after morning transfusion	Maximizes safety

Category	Subcategory	Details/Guidelines	Clinical Notes
INR Requirement	Acceptable Level	INR ≤ 3.5	Safe for most invasive dental procedures
Liver Disease Coagulation	Bleeding vs Clotting	Risk of both bleeding and hypercoagulability	Complex haemostasis
	Complication	Risk of Deep Vein Thrombosis	Can be emergency
Alcohol History	Assessment	Type, frequency, duration	Important for liver evaluation
Oral Signs	Findings	Poor dental health, xerostomia, mucosal jaundice	Common in liver disease
Systemic Signs	Findings	Malnutrition, spider angiomas, palmar erythema	Clinical indicators
	Advanced Signs	Ascites, splenomegaly	Suggest chronic liver disease

1. Alcoholic Liver Disease & Cirrhosis

Alcoholic liver disease (ALD) results from chronic, excessive alcohol consumption, which leads to progressive hepatocellular injury and death.

- In the early stages, liver damage is reversible if alcohol intake ceases.
- Continued alcohol consumption results in a predictable progression:
    1. Fatty liver (hepatic steatosis)
    2. Alcoholic hepatitis
    3. Alcoholic cirrhosis (irreversible)

Table 4-3: Dental & Anaesthetic Considerations in Alcoholic Cirrhosis

Category	Subcategory	Details/Guidelines	Clinical Notes
Drug Response	Increased Tolerance	Higher tolerance to local anaesthetics, hypnotics, sedatives	May require higher doses cautiously
Local Anaesthesia	Requirement	Adjust dose based on response	Avoid overdose due to impaired metabolism
Sedation	Response	Reduced sensitivity to sedatives	Careful titration needed
Invasive Procedures	Suitability	May be contraindicated	Depends on severity
Pre-procedure Assessment	Bleeding Risk	Evaluate platelet count, INR	High risk in cirrhosis
	Liver Function	Assess severity of disease	Impacts drug metabolism
	Coordination	Physician consultation	Essential before invasive care

2. Hepatitis B

Table 4-4: Dental Drug–Hepatitis B Drug Interactions

Category	Dental Drug	Hepatitis B Drug	Interaction/ Risk	Management
NSAIDs & Analgesics	Ibuprofen/ Ibuprofen–hydrocodone/ Naproxen	Telbivudine	↑ Kidney dysfunction, ↑ telbivudine levels	Physician consult, dose adjustment, monitor
	Aspirin/ Aspirin–oxycodone	Telbivudine	↑ Risk of adverse effects	Avoid or use cautiously; consult physician

Category	Dental Drug	Hepatitis B Drug	Interaction/ Risk	Management
Antibiotics	Metronidazole	Telbivudine, Interferon alfa-2b	↑ Risk of neuropathy	Dose adjustment; mandatory consultation
Corticosteroids	Prednisone/ Hydrocortisone	Telbivudine	↑ Risk of muscle disorders	Physician consultation required
Opioids/ Combination Analgesics	Tramadol/ Tramadol–acetaminophen	Interferon alfa-2b, Pegylated interferon	↑ Seizure risk	Avoid or consult physician

Dental notes: Patients with active hepatitis B infection

- Even though the dental professional has been vaccinated against HCB, the seroconversion (development of detectable antibodies) risk is 30%.
- Use universal infection control methods.

3. Hepatitis C

Table 4-5: Dental considerations in patients with Hepatitis C

Category	Subcategory	Details/Guidelines	Clinical Notes
Medical Consultation	Physician Coordination	Mandatory consultation	Essential before dental treatment
	Laboratory Tests	CBC with WBC differential & platelet count	Assess infection & bleeding risk
	Risk Assessment	Evaluate bleeding & infection risk	Before invasive procedures
Oral Manifestations	Oral Lichen Planus	Strong independent association with Hepatitis C	Occurs even without medication

(Contd.)

Category	Subcategory	Details/Guidelines	Clinical Notes
Drug Therapy Effects	Treatment	Interferon + Ribavirin therapy	Common antiviral regimen
	Oral Reactions	Lichen planus, aphthous ulcers	Mucosal involvement
	Pigmentation	Tongue & skin hyperpigmentation	Drug-related effect
	Systemic Reaction	Systemic Lupus Erythematosus	Rare but significant
Timing of Adverse Effects	Early Onset	Within ~3 days of therapy	Acute reactions
	Delayed Onset	≥ 3 days after starting therapy	Monitor continuously

- Always consult physician + check CBC
- Watch for lichen planus (strong association)
- Antiviral therapy → multiple oral & systemic adverse effects
- Reactions may be early or delayed → continuous monitoring needed

4. Liver Transplant Patients

Table 4-6 : Dental Drug–Drug Interactions in Liver Transplant Patients

Category	Dental Drug	Interacts With	Interaction/Risk	Management
Macrolide Antibiotics	Clarithromycin/ Erythromycin	Cyclosporine, Tacrolimus	↑ Immunosuppressant levels → toxicity; QT prolongation	Avoid; prefer azithromycin or clindamycin
Fluoroquinolones	Ciprofloxacin	Cyclosporine	↑ Cyclosporine levels → nephrotoxicity	Avoid
Lincosamides	Clindamycin	Mycophenolate	↓ Mycophenolate levels	Use with caution

Category	Dental Drug	Interacts With	Interaction/Risk	Management
Azole Antifungals	Fluconazole/ Ketoconazole/ Clotrimazole	Cyclosporine, Tacrolimus, Sirolimus	↑ Immunosuppressant levels → nephrotoxicity, neurotoxicity	Consult physician; dose reduction may be needed
	Azoles + Statins	Atorvastatin, Simvastatin, Lovastatin	↑ Statin toxicity (CYP3A4 inhibition)	Avoid combination
Corticosteroids	Prednisone/ others	Cyclosporine, Tacrolimus, Sirolimus	↑ Risk of adrenal suppression, toxicity	Avoid if possible; consult nephrologist
	Corticosteroids + Mycophenolate	Mycophenolate	↑ Immunosuppression & infection risk	Use cautiously
Other Antibiotics	Metronidazole	Mycophenolate	↑ Drug levels	Use with caution
	Tetracycline	Mycophenolate	↓ Drug levels	Monitor
	Azithromycin/ Clarithromycin/ Erythromycin	Mycophenolate	↓ Drug levels	Use cautiously
Antivirals	Acyclovir/ Valacyclovir	Mycophenolate	↑ Toxicity of both drugs	Monitor closely

Liver Transplant Patient:

Medical Consultation

- Physician consultation is mandatory
- Required to determine:
  - Need for antibiotic prophylaxis
  - Bleeding risk
  - Status of immunosuppression
- Obtain a current CBC with differential

Antibiotic Prophylaxis

- No universal protocol
- Consult the patient's physician/transplant team before prescribing
- May be required depending on:
  - Immune status
  - Presence of infection
  - Type of dental procedure

Management of Oral Infections

- Active oral infections must be eliminated
  - Treat dental caries
  - Drain abscesses
  - Manage periodontal disease
- Non-restorable teeth should be extracted
- Post-operative antibiotics may be required to prevent systemic infection

Oral Hygiene

- Review and reinforce oral hygiene home-care instructions
- Emphasize:
  - Pre-transplantation dental care
  - Post-transplantation maintenance to reduce infection risk

Medication Review

- Instruct patient to bring a written list of all medications at every dental visit
- Be aware that patients are commonly on:
  - Immunosuppressive drugs (e.g., cyclosporine, tacrolimus, mycophenolate)

Infection Risk

- Post-transplant infection is the leading cause of organ rejection
- Strict:
  - Infection control
  - Aseptic technique
  - Early management of oral disease

Bleeding Tendencies

- Physician consultation required
- Obtain:
  - Recent platelet count
  - CBC with differential
- Many patients may have:
  - Thrombocytopenia (<50,000/mm^3)
    - May require platelet transfusion
    - Transfusion is typically done the morning of dental extraction
- If on anticoagulants (e.g., warfarin):
  - Obtain INR within 24 hours (not more than 72 hours) before the procedure.

5. Gall Stones

- There are no specific dental management problems with patients with gallstones.
- Some risk factors that can be monitored in the dental office include smoking, heavy drinking, diabetes, and imbalanced diet.

References

Bernard, B., Grange, J.D., Khac, E.N., *et al.* (1999) Antibiotic prophylaxis for the prevention of bacterial infections in cirrhotic patients with gastrointestinal bleeding: a meta-analysis. *Hepatology*, 29, 1655–1661.

Byron, R.J. Jr. & Osborne, P.D. (2005) Dental management of liver transplant patients. *General Dentistry*, 53, 66–69.

Douglas, L.R., Douglass, J.B., Sieck, J.O., *et al.* (1998) Oral management of the patient with end-stage liver disease and the liver transplant patient. *Oral Surgery Oral Medicine Oral Pathology Oral Radiology, and Endodontology*, 86, 55–64.

Golla, K., Epstein, J.B., & Cabay, R.J. (2004) Liver disease: current perspectives on medical and dental management. *Oral Surgery Oral Medicine Oral Pathology Oral Radiology, and Endodontology*, 98, 516–521.

Grossman S. M., Teixeira, R., de Aguiar, M.C., *et al.* (2009) Oral mucosal conditions in chronic hepatitis C.

Guggenheimer, J., Eghtesad, B., & Stock, D.J. (2003) Dental management of the (solid) organ transplant patient. *Oral Surgery Oral Medicine Oral Pathology Oral Radiology and Endodontology*, 95, 383–389.

Little, J.W., Falace, D.A., Miller, C.S. *et al.* (2008) Liver disease. In: J.W. Little, D.A. Falace, C.S. Miller, et al. (eds), *Dental Management of the Medically Compromised Patient*, 7th edn, pp. 140–161. Mosby Elsevier, St. Louis, MO.

Pamplona, M.C., Munoz, M.M., & Perez, M.C.S. (2011) Dental considerations in patients with liver disease. *Journal Clinical Experimental Dentistry*, 3 (2), e127–e134.

Smith, A.J., Cameron, S.O., Bagg, J., *et al.* (2001) Management of needlestick injuries in general dental practice. *British Dental Journal*, 190, 645–650.

Smith, E. & Desmond, P. (2013) Prescribing in patients with abnormal liver function tests. *Australian Family Physician*, 42, 30–33.

Strader, D.B., Wright, T., Thomas, D.L., *et al.* (2004) American Association for the Study of Liver Diseases. Diagnosis, management, and treatment of hepatitis C. *Hepatology*, 39 (4), 1147–1171.

Williford, S.K., Salisbury, P.L., Peacock, J.E. *et al.* (1989) The safety of dental extractions in patients with hematologic malignancies. *Journal of Clinical Oncology*, 7, 798–802.

Chapter 5

Dental Management of Diabetic Patients

Introduction

Dental management of diabetic patients requires careful monitoring of blood glucose levels, optimizing metabolic control, and managing risks of infection and hypoglycaemia. Early morning appointments are preferred to minimize stress and prevent hypoglycaemia. Key strategies include consulting physicians for poor control, using chairside blood glucose monitoring, prophylactic antibiotics for surgical procedures to prevent delayed healing, and managing oral complications like periodontitis.

Dental Management of Diabetic Patients

I. Oral adverse effects of diabetes

- Periodontal Disease: Higher risk due to impaired immunity and vascular changes.
- Xerostomia: Dry mouth increases risk of dental caries.
- Glossitis: Inflammation or soreness of the tongue.
- Burning Mouth Syndrome
- Candidiasis: Fungal infections from decreased salivary flow and high glucose levels.

II. Dental Management Guidelines

Before the Appointment

- Review full medical and medication history (antihypertensives, statins, insulin/oral agents).
- Ask if the patient:
  - Took their insulin or oral hypoglycaemic medication that day.
  - Monitored their blood glucose levels (ask for the result).
  - Has a history of hypoglycaemic reactions.

During the Appointment

- Monitor blood pressure at each visit due to cardiovascular risks.
- Screen and monitor for periodontal disease.
- Educate on the bidirectional link between diabetes and gum disease.
- Observe for signs of:
  - Xerostomia
  - Burning mouth
  - Candidiasis

In Case of Hypoglycaemia

- If conscious: Give sugar, orange juice, or glucose tablets.
- If unconscious: Call emergency services. Administer glucagon or IV dextrose.

III. Drug Interactions to Watch For

Table 5-1: Effect and management of drugs in diabetic patients

Drug	Effect	Management
Aspirin/NSAIDs	↑ Insulin effect → hypoglycaemia	Use caution
Systemic corticosteroids	↑ Blood glucose	May need dose adjustment; consult physician

(Contd.)

Drug	Effect	Management
Azole antifungals (e.g., fluconazole)	May cause acute hypoglycaemia	Space medicines 2 hrs apart
Fluoroquinolones (e.g., ciprofloxacin)	Can impair insulin/ glucose balance	Use alternatives or monitor

IV. Local Anaesthetic Use

- Epinephrine is safe in most diabetics.
- Avoid in unmedicated or uncontrolled diabetics due to risk of epinephrine-induced hyperglycaemia.
- No correlation found between number of cartridges and glucose changes.

V. Glycaemic Control Goals

- HbA1c Targets: For extractions, dental implants and other surgical procedures
  - AACE: <6.5%
  - ADA: <7.0%

VI. Additional Notes

- Low-dose aspirin (75–162 mg/day) is recommended for secondary prevention in diabetics with a history of cardiovascular disease.
- Comprehensive oral exams and preventive care are key for maintaining oral and systemic health in diabetic patients.

Always document blood glucose readings, medical history updates in the dental chart.

References

The Dentist's Quick Guide to Medical Conditions, First Edition. Mea A. Weinberg, Stuart L. Segelnick, Joseph S. Insler, with Samuel Kramer. 2015 John Wiley & Sons, Inc. Published 2015 by John Wiley & Sons, Inc.

Chapter 6

Dental Management of Thyroid Disorders

Introduction

Dental management of thyroid disorders requires a thorough medical history check to confirm stability and prevent emergencies like thyroid storms. Uncontrolled hyperthyroidism and hypothyroidism require delaying elective procedures, while controlled patients typically receive standard care with precautions regarding epinephrine usage and potential medication interactions.

Oral Manifestations and Dental Management of Thyroid Disorders:

Table 6-1: Oral Aspects and management for thyroid disorders

Category	Hypothyroidism	Hyperthyroidism
Oral Manifestations	• Delayed tooth eruption • Delayed wound healing • Enamel hypoplasia • Mouth breathing • Glossitis • Salivary gland enlargement Dysgeusia • Anterior open bite • Macroglossia	• Periodontal disease • Increased dental caries • Burning mouth syndrome • Accelerated tooth eruption • Possible association with autoimmune conditions (e.g., Sjögren's, SLE)

(Contd.)

Category	Hypothyroidism	Hyperthyroidism
Wound Healing	Delayed healing; ↑ infection risk	Usually normal (unless severe/ uncontrolled)
Tooth Eruption	Delayed	Accelerated
Caries Risk	Normal to slightly increased	Increased
Periodontal Risk	Possibly increased (due to impaired healing)	Increased
Systemic/ Special Considerations	• Increased risk of cardiovascular disease • May be on anticoagulants (e.g., Warfarin). Avoid NSAIDs/aspirin if on anticoagulants • Consider medical consult if undiagnosed or poorly controlled	• Reduce stress/anxiety (risk of crisis) Monitor vital signs • Limit epinephrine (≤2 cartridges of 1:80,000). • Avoid treatment in uncontrolled state (risk of thyroid storm)
Dental Drug Considerations	Increased sensitivity to CNS depressants (use cautiously). Monitor vital signs	Avoid excessive epinephrine; caution with stimulants
Emergency Risk	Myxoedema coma (rare)	Thyroid storm (life-threatening)
Referral Criteria	Undiagnosed symptoms or poor control → medical consult	Undiagnosed symptoms or poor control → medical consult

References

The Dentist's Quick Guide to Medical Conditions, First Edition. Mea A. Weinberg, Stuart L. Segelnick, Joseph S. Insler, with Samuel Kramer. 2015 John Wiley & Sons, Inc. Published 2015 by John Wiley & Sons, Inc.

Chapter 7

Guidelines for Patients Taking Systemic Corticosteroids

Introduction

Dental management of patients on systemic corticosteroids requires assessing for adrenal insufficiency and infection risk. For stressful procedures, patients may need supplementary doses to prevent adrenal crisis. Monitor closely for delayed healing and oral candidiasis, and consider topical alternatives when possible.

Adrenal Corticosteroids – Clinical Overview

Functions & Uses

Adrenal corticosteroids are used for:

- Replacement therapy
    - Adrenal insufficiency
    - Hypopituitarism
    - Congenital adrenal hyperplasia
- Therapeutic effects
    - Anti-inflammatory
    - Immunosuppressive

- Common conditions treated
  - Asthma
  - Rheumatoid arthritis
  - Nephrotic syndrome
  - Autoimmune diseases (SLE, pemphigus)
  - Severe allergies
  - Organ transplant rejection

Adrenal Gland Structure & Hormones

1. Adrenal Medulla

- Produces:
  - Epinephrine
  - Norepinephrine
- Function:
  - Activates sympathetic nervous system
  - Causes glycogenolysis → ↑ blood glucose

2. Adrenal Cortex

Produces steroid hormones from cholesterol.

Control Mechanism:

- Hypothalamus → Pituitary → ACTH
- ACTH stimulates corticosteroid release

Types of Adrenal Corticosteroids

1. Mineralocorticoids

- Main hormone: Aldosterone
- Function:
  - Regulate fluid & electrolyte balance
  - ↑ Sodium retention

    - ↑ Potassium excretion
    - Maintain blood pressure (via renin–angiotensin system)
- Clinical use:
    - Hypoadrenalism
- Example:
    - Fludrocortisone

2. Glucocorticoids

Primary hormone:

- Cortisol (Hydrocortisone)

Functions:

- Metabolic:
    - Protein breakdown → glucose
    - Fat breakdown → glucose
    - Glycogen to glucose

      (Gluconeogenesis + Glycogenolysis)
- Anti-inflammatory
- Anti-allergic
- Immunosuppressive

Potency Equivalents:

Drug	Equivalent Dose
Hydrocortisone	20 mg
Prednisone	5 mg
Dexamethasone	0.75 mg

Normal & Stress Secretion:

- Normal: 20–30 mg/day cortisol
- Minor stress: ~50 mg/day

- Major surgery: 75–150 mg/day
- Severe stress: up to 300 mg/day

3. Gonadocorticoids

- Produced by adrenal cortex (minor role)
- Include:
  - Androgens (testosterone)
  - Oestrogen
  - Progesterone
- Supplement gonadal hormones

Mechanism of Action (Glucocorticoids)

- Enter cells → bind intracellular receptors
- Regulate gene transcription
- Control protein synthesis

Effects:

- ↓ Inflammatory mediators
- ↓ Histamine release (mast cells)
- ↓ Immune response

Diagnostic/Lab Values

- Cortisol measurement (plasma/urine) used for diagnosis

Circadian Rhythm:

- Morning → High cortisol
- Evening → Low cortisol

Stress Effect:

- Stress overrides circadian rhythm
- ↑ ACTH → ↑ cortisol production

Table 7-1: Corticosteroids: Adverse Effects & Dental Management

Aspect	Details	Dental Implications/ Management
Steroid-induced diabetes	↑ Blood glucose with long-term use	Monitor blood sugar, ↑ risk of periodontal disease, delayed healing
Adrenal suppression	↓ Endogenous cortisol due to exogenous steroids	Risk of adrenal crisis during stress → assess history carefully
Adrenal crisis	Hypotension, weakness, abdominal pain, nausea, vomiting	Medical emergency; rare in dentistry; prevent with stress reduction
Minor dental procedures (LA)	Routine procedures, simple extraction	No steroid supplementation if <7.5 mg prednisone/day
Major procedures (GA)	Extensive oral/ periodontal surgery	May need steroid supplementation (double dose); medical consult required
High-dose steroid therapy	Long-term high-dose systemic steroids	↑ Risk of adrenal suppression → consider supplementation
Low-risk patients	Inhaled steroids, alternate-day therapy, ≤5 mg/day	No supplementation needed
Dose equivalence	20 mg hydrocortisone = 5 mg prednisone = 0.75 mg dexamethasone	Helps assess adequacy of steroid coverage
Stress response	Cortisol ↑ up to 300 mg/ day in stress	Do not exceed this level when supplementing
Appointment timing	Morning appointments	Cortisol levels highest → safer
Pre-op preparation	Take steroid within 2 hours	Ensures adequate circulating cortisol
Stress reduction	Anxiety control, profound anaesthesia	Prevents adrenal crisis

(Contd.)

Aspect	Details	Dental Implications/ Management
Local anaesthesia	Use long-acting LA, adequate analgesia	Reduces procedural stress
Drug interactions	NSAIDs & aspirin	Avoid → risk of gastric ulcer/ bleeding
Epinephrine use	From adrenal medulla	Safe to use
Monitoring	Blood pressure	Check before & after procedure
When to refer	Suspected adrenal insufficiency	Refer to endocrinologist

Table 7-2: Risk categories and considerations in patients on corticosteroids

Risk Category	Dental Procedure	Target Steroid Level	Supplemental Steroids Required	Additional Notes
Low Risk	Minor nonsurgical procedures without local anaesthetic	~5 mg prednisone	No – continue regular steroid dose	No supplemental dose needed
Mild Risk	Minor periodontal/ oral surgery with local anaesthetic (e.g., single extraction, SRP)	~5–6 mg prednisone (≈25 mg hydrocortisone/ day)	No – continue regular steroid dose	Take 1–2 hours before treatment
Moderate to Major Risk	Major oral surgery or extensive procedures	50–100 mg hydrocortisone/ day	Yes – increase dose or administer IM hydrocortisone	Consult physician; analgesics as needed

Risk Category	**Dental Procedure**	**Target Steroid Level**	**Supplemental Steroids Required**	**Additional Notes**
			Option 1: 100 mg IM hydrocortisone 1 hour prior	
			Option 2: Double usual 5 mg prednisone to 10 mg 2 hrs before, then 10 mg next day	Resume normal dosing after one day

References

The Dentist's Quick Guide to Medical Conditions, First Edition. Mea A. Weinberg, Stuart L. Segelnick, Joseph S. Insler, with Samuel Kramer. 2015 John Wiley & Sons, Inc. Published 2015 by John Wiley & Sons, Inc.

Chapter 8

Dental Management of the Hypertensive Patient & Cardiac Disorders

Introduction

Dental management for hypertensive and cardiac patients focuses on risk assessment, stress reduction, and careful medication use to prevent adverse events like stroke or myocardial infarction (MI).

Management of Hypertensive patient

Table 8-1: Interactions and side effects of various Hypertensive drugs

Drug Class	NSAID Interaction	Orthostatic Hypotension	Xerostomia	Epinephrine Precautions	Other Notes
Diuretics	↓ Effectiveness (↑ BP)	Monitor closely	Yes	None	Increased urination – time appointments accordingly
ACE Inhibitors	↓ Effectiveness (↑ BP)	Monitor closely	Yes	None	—
ARBs	↓ Effectiveness (↑ BP)	Monitor closely	Yes	None	—

Drug Class	NSAID Interaction	Orthostatic Hypotension	Xerostomia	Epinephrine Precautions	Other Notes
Central α_2-Adrenergic Inhibitors	Least affected	Monitor closely	Yes	None	—
Peripheral Adrenergic Inhibitors	↓ Effectiveness (↑ BP)	Monitor closely	Yes	None	—
β_1-Blockers (Vasodilating)	↓ Effectiveness (↑ BP)	Monitor closely	Yes	None	—
β-Blockers (Non-selective)	↓ Effectiveness (↑ BP)	Monitor closely	Yes	Limit epinephrine: (Use minimal amount of epinephrine (two cartrides 1:100,000) for Labetalol, Nadolol, Propranolol	Others: no epinephrine precautions
CCBs (Calcium Channel Blockers)	No interaction	Monitor closely	Yes	None	Gingival enlargement (esp. nifedipine, amlodipine)
Direct Vasodilators	↓ Effectiveness (↑ BP)	Monitor closely	Yes	None	—

Dental Management of the Hypertensive Patient

1. Blood Pressure Guidelines for Dental Treatment

Table 8-2: Dental considerations based on BP Reading

BP Reading (mmHg)	Dental Treatment Guidance
≤ 140/90	Proceed with treatment as normal
141–159/91–95	Proceed with caution; monitor vitals frequently
≥ 160/95	Delay non-emergency dental care; consult physician
≥ 180/110	DO NOT TREAT; recheck BP after 5 mins rest. If still elevated, seek emergency medical care

2. Pre-Treatment Considerations

- Confirm medications taken that day; if not taken, postpone treatment.
- Always update the medical history.
- Ask about last physician visit and usual BP.
- Discuss the condition the antihypertensive medications are treating.
- Consult physician for uncontrolled BP or complex medication regimens.
- Smoking cessation should be included in the care plan.

3. In-Treatment Considerations

- Take and document BP multiple times during treatment.
- Appointments should be short, morning sessions to reduce stress.
- Consider nitrous oxide or benzodiazepines to reduce anxiety.
- Let the patient sit upright for a few minutes post-procedure to prevent orthostatic hypotension.

4. Medication side effects

- ACE Inhibitors (ACEIs):

    - May cause angioedema of lips/tongue—refer to physician.
    - Can cause oral lichenoid reactions or lichen planus–like lesions.
- Thiazide diuretics:
    - Also associated with oral lichenoid reactions.
    - Can contribute to xerostomia—manage with hydration, avoid alcohol-based rinses, and apply fluoride.
- NSAIDs + Antihypertensives:
    - Avoid NSAIDs (e.g., ibuprofen, naproxen) >5 days as they reduce efficacy of antihypertensive drugs (except CCBs).
- CCBs (e.g., Nifedipine):
    - Commonly cause gingival enlargement; manage with home care or surgical intervention; may reverse with drug discontinuation.

5. Vasoconstrictors and Anaesthesia

Table 8-3: Vasoconstrictor guidelines for High BP patients

Vasoconstrictor Use	Guideline
Epinephrine 1:100,000	Safe for most; limit to 2 cartridges (0.034 mg) in cardiovascular patients
1:50,000 epinephrine or retraction cords with epi	Avoid in hypertensive patients
Levonordefrin (α-agonist in mepivacaine)	Avoid in hypertensive patients
Nonselective β-blockers (e.g., propranolol)	Use minimum epinephrine dose (½ cartridge); monitor closely

- Always aspirate to avoid intravascular injection.
- Monitor for toxicity: increased BP, tachycardia, arrhythmias.
- BP can be taken after injection if necessary.

6. Special BP Monitoring Sites

- Post-mastectomy or lymph node removal: Avoid affected arm. Use leg or ankle (popliteal artery) if needed.
- Morbid obesity: Use popliteal artery or thigh cuff for accuracy.

7. Medication Considerations

Table 8-4: Drug class and oral effects

Drug Class	Potential Oral Effects/Notes
ACE Inhibitors	Angioedema (lips/tongue); oral lichenoid reactions; consult physician if swelling occurs
Thiazide Diuretics	Oral lichenoid reactions, xerostomia
CCBs (e.g., Nifedipine)	Gingival enlargement—reversible with discontinuation
All Antihypertensives	May cause orthostatic hypotension—sit patient up slowly post-treatment
NSAID Interaction	Avoid >5 days with all antihypertensives except CCBs—reduces antihypertensive efect

8. Additional Clinical Tips

Table 8-5: Dental considerations in different situations

Situation	Action
Missed BP meds day of appointment	Postpone treatment
High anxiety	Consider nitrous oxide or benzodiazepine (short-term)
After mastectomy or lymph node removal	Use opposite arm or leg (above knee) for BP
Morbidly obese	Use popliteal artery (ankle/thigh) for BP
Xerostomia management	Hydration, avoid alcohol rinses, use fluoride/ remineralizing agents
Smoking	Integrate smoking cessation into treatment plan

DENTAL MANAGEMENT OF PATIENTS WITH ANGINA

Table 8-6: Dental Management of Patients with Angina – Clinical Reference Chart

Category	Recommendations
Assessment & History	• Assess severity and stability of angina • Inquire about last attack, triggers, and relief measures • Confirm use of nitroglycerin and other medications
Before Appointment	• Ensure nitroglycerin is available in operatory • Patient should bring own nitroglycerin
If Chest Pain Occurs	1. Stop all dental procedures 2. Have patient rest and take nitroglycerin 3. Wait a few minutes and monitor BP and HR 4. Administer oxygen as needed
Chair Positioning	• Risk of orthostatic hypotension with nitrates • Have patient sit upright for a few minutes before standing
Local Anaesthesia	• Stable angina: Use max 2 cartridges of 1:100,000 epinephrine • Alternative: 1:200,000 epinephrine (e.g., 4% articaine) • Helps achieve profound anaesthesia and reduce stress
Sedation & Appointment	• Consider short appointments • Mild/moderate (conscious) sedation may be indicated
Aspirin Use	• Do not discontinue aspirin for routine periodontal debridement
Epinephrine Use	• Safe in stable angina patients • No special precautions required if angina is stable
Elective Dentistry	• Postpone if patient has unstable angina

Table 8-7: Dental management of patients on antianginal drugs:

Drug Class	Examples	Mechanism of Action	Dental Management
Nitrates	Nitroglycerin	Dilates and relaxes coronary blood vessels	Headache, dizziness, flushing, orthostatic hypotension. Monitor BP. Allow patient to sit upright in dental chair before dismissal.
	Isosorbidedinitrate	Same	No special precautions with epinephrine.
Calcium Channel Blockers	Amlodipine, Bedpridil, Diltiazem,	Slows heart rate and dilates coronary arteries	Orthostatic hypotension: Allow upright sitting before dismissal. Nifedipine may cause gingival enlargement. No special precautions with epinephrine.
	Nifedipine, Verapamil		
Cardioselective Beta-Blockers (β_1)	Atenolol, Metoprolol	Reduces cardiac load and oxygen demand	NSAIDs like naproxen sodium and ibuprofen may decrease antihypertensive effects → possible rapid BP elevation.
Non-cardioselective Beta-Blockers	Nadolol	Affects both β_1 and β_2 receptors	Orthostatic hypotension: Monitor BP. Let patient sit upright before leaving.
	Propranolol	Same	No epinephrine use (risk of hypertensive reaction).

DENTAL MANAGEMENT OF MI PATIENT

Table 8-8: Medication management of the MI dental patient

Category	Guideline
Medical Consult	Always required before initiating treatment
Post-MI Treatment Timing	No treatment within first 30 days- Ideally delay treatment for 6 months- Treatment may be considered after 3 months
Post-CABG Treatment Timing	Delay dental treatment for 3 months
Monitoring	Monitor blood pressure and heart rate at every appointment
Epinephrine Use	Limit to 2 cartridges of 1:100,000 epinephrine
Appointment Modifications	Keep appointments short and apply stress-reduction techniques
Antibiotic Prophylaxis	Not required for patients with coronary stents
Analgesics (with Warfarin)	Avoid aspirin and NSAIDs (ibuprofen, naproxen)- may raise INR- Use hydrocodone short-term- Prefer Regular Paracetamol
NSAID Risks (General)	NSAIDs increase CV risk and mortality post-MI; no safe treatment window
Emergency Protocol (Suspected MI)	- Call EMS- Lay patient supine- Assess ABCs (Airway, Breathing, Circulation)- Monitor vital signs

Table 8-9: International Normalized Ratio (INR) Guidelines for Dental Treatment

Condition	Acceptable INR Range	Notes
All patients (general rule)	< 4.0	INR must be under 4.0 for dental procedures
Pulmonary embolism (PE)	2.0 – 3.0	
Deep vein thrombosis (DVT)	2.0 – 3.0	
Atrial fibrillation (AF)	2.0 – 3.0	
Bileaflet mitral valve	2.0 – 3.0	
Mechanical heart valves	3.0 – 4.0	Higher target INR due to thrombosis risk
Recurrent embolism while on warfarin	3.0 – 4.0	Indicates warfarin resistance or higher clotting risk

Dental Management Notes

- Check INR within 24–72 hours prior to invasive procedures.
- Do not discontinue warfarin without medical consultation.
- Routine dental work is typically safe within the target INR ranges.

Epinephrine in cardiac patients

Low-Dose Epinephrine (0.18 mg, ~1–2 dental cartridges)

- Receptor Affinity:
  - β2-receptors have a higher affinity for epinephrine than α-receptors.
- Effect at Low Dose:
  - Primarily β2 stimulation → vasodilation in skeletal muscle vasculature.

- Hemodynamic Outcome:
  - ↓ Diastolic BP (due to vasodilation)
  - ↑ Systolic BP (mild due to cardiac stimulation)
  - Mean arterial pressure stays relatively stable
- Clinical Relevance:

Inject slowly and aspirate to prevent intravascular injection and exaggerated systemic effects.

High-Dose Epinephrine (0.5–1 mg, emergency use)

- Receptor Activation:
  - α-receptor stimulation → vasoconstriction (dominant effect)
  - Followed by β1 stimulation → increased heart rate and contractility
- Hemodynamic Outcome:
  - ↑ Systolic and Diastolic BP
- Use Cases:
  - Anaphylaxis
  - Cardiac arrest

Key Takeaways

- Epinephrine's receptor selectivity depends on the dose.
- Low doses: Favor β2 effects → vasodilation, decreased diastolic pressure.
- High doses: Favor α and β1 effects → vasoconstriction, increased BP and cardiac output.
- Clinical caution: Always inject dental anesthetics with epinephrine slowly and aspirate to avoid systemic complications.

Table 8-10 : Timing of Dental Treatment Following Cardiac Procedures

Cardiac Procedure	**Recommended Timing to Initiate Dental Treatment**
Coronary artery bypass graft (CABG)	After 6 months; no antibiotic premedication required
Pacemaker	Dental treatment may be initiated within the first few weeks; no antibiotic premedication required
Cardiac stent	After 3 months; generally, no antibiotic premedication required
Angioplasty or cardiac catheterization	No need to postpone dental treatment; no antibiotic premedication required
Artificial valves or shunts	Minimum of 3 months; antibiotic prophylaxis required
Myocardial infarction	Minimum of 6 months; no antibiotic premedication required

References

American Academy of Periodontology (1996) Periodontal management of patients with cardiovascular diseases. *Journal of Periodontology*, 67, 627–635.

Ardekian, L., Gaspar, R., Peled, M., *et al.* (2000) Does low-dose aspirin therapy complicate oral surgical procedures? *The Journal of the American Dental Association*, 131, 331–335.

Bader, J.D., Bonito, A.U., & Shugars, D.A. (2002) A systematic review of cardiovascular effects of epinephrine on hypertensive dental patients. *Oral Surgery Oral Medicine Oral Pathology Oral Radiology Endodontics*, 93, 647–653.

Bradley, J.G. & Davis, K.A. (2003) Orthostatic hypotension. *American Family Physician* 68, 2398–2398.

Hersh, E.V. & Moore, P.A. (2008) Adverse drug interactions in dentistry. *Periodontology* 2000, 46, 109–142.

Jeske, A.H. & Suchko, G.D. (2003) Lack of a scientific basis for routine discontinuation of oral anticoagulation therapy before dental treatment. *The Journal of the American Dental Association*, 134, 1492–1497.

Karp, J.M. & Moss, A.J. (2006) Dental treatment of patients with long QT syndrome. *Journal of the American Dental Association*, 137, 630–637.

Lifshey, F.M. (2004) Evaluation of and treatment considerations for the dental patient with cardiac disease. *New York State Dental Journal*, 70, 16–19.

Nichols, C. (1997) Dentistry and hypertension. *Journal of the American Dental Association*, 128, 1557–1562.

Perusse, R., Goulet J.-P., & Turcotte, J.-Y. (1992) Contraindications to vasoconstrictors in dentistry. Part I. *Oral Surgery Oral Medicine Oral Pathology*, 74, 679–786.

Schmelzeisen, R., Yabroudi, F., & Dannan, A. (2009) Pre-and post-operative dental focus of patients with prosthetic heart valves. *The Internet Journal of Cardiovascular Research*, 6 (1), 2–3. DOI:10.5580/1fe0.

Skaar, D., O'Connor, H., Lunos, S., *et al.* (2012) Dental procedures and risk of experiencing a second vascular event in a Medicare population. *Journal of the American Medical Association*, 143, 1190–1198.

Chapter 9

Dental Management of Bleeding Disorders & those taking Anticoagulation Medications

Introduction

Dental management for patients with bleeding disorders or those on anticoagulants focuses on balancing the risk of bleeding from procedures against the risk of thromboembolic events (like stroke or heart attack) if medications are stopped. Most minor dental procedures can be safely performed without altering or interrupting medication, provided that effective local haemostatic measures are used.

Pre-Treatment Considerations

1. Medical Consultation:
   - Obtain recent CBC, clotting profile, and consult the patient's physician.
2. Patient History:
   - Review medical and family history for:
     - Epistaxis (nosebleeds)
     - Spontaneous gingival bleeding
     - Prolonged post-extraction bleeding
     - Family members with bleeding disorders

3. Medication Review:
    - Pay attention to aspirin (even low dose) and anticoagulants.
4. Clinical Signs:
    - Petechiae, ecchymoses, hematomas, or spontaneous gingival bleeding → suspect bleeding disorder and refer.
5. Setting of Care:
    - Decide between office vs. hospital setting (especially for general anaesthesia cases).

Bleeding Disorders Classification

Coagulation Disorders (e.g., Haemophilia, von Willebrand Disease)

- Treatment varies by type of disorder and severity (e.g., vWD Type I/II/III).

Platelet Disorders (Eg; ITP, Liver disorders)

- >50,000 platelets/mm^3: Usually safe for surgical procedures.
- <10,000–20,000: Risk of spontaneous bleeding.
- <50,000: Transfusion usually required (1 unit ↑ ~6,000 platelets; often 6 units used).
    - Reversible thrombocytopenia: Postpone elective dental care until recovery.
    - Irreversible thrombocytopenia: Require transfusion pre-procedure.

Table 9-1: Medical/Drug Management of Patients with Bleeding Disorders

Bleeding Disorder	**Management**
Thrombocytopenia	Consult haematologist • Check platelet count ≥2 days before procedure • Delay if < 50,000/μL • Transfuse on morning of procedure if needed • Use haemostatic agents, antifibrinolytic rinses • Avoid aspirin and NSAIDs

(Contd.)

Bleeding Disorder	Management
von Willebrand Disease	• Consult haematologist - Use DDAVP/factor VIII replacement - Local haemostatic measures - Use haemostatic agents - Avoid aspirin and NSAIDs
Haemophilia	• Consult haematologist - Haemophilia A: increase factor VIII (recombinant/plasma-derived) - DDAVP for mild Haemophilia A - Antifibrinolytics (e.g., E-aminocaproic acid) - Use good surgical technique, sutures - Avoid aspirin and NSAIDs
Severe Liver Disease	• Consult hepatologist - Platelet count, INR may guide transfusion - Use acetaminophen cautiously - Avoid aspirin and NSAIDs
Antiplatelet Drugs (Aspirin, Clopidogrel/ Plavix, Ticlopidine, Prasugrel, Abciximab, Dipyridamole)	• INR not useful for bleeding risk - Avoid aspirin and NSAIDs - Use pressure until haemostasis is achieved
Anticoagulant Drugs(Warfarin, Apixaban, Dabigatran, Rivaroxaban)	• Warfarin: INR within 24–72 h before procedure - Obtain primary closure - NO INR needed for Apixaban, Dabigatran, Rivaroxaban - Use local haemostatic measures (pressure with gauze) - Avoid aspirin and NSAIDs

Table 9-2: Management of Patients with Bleeding Disorders based on dental procedure to be done

Dental Procedure	Management Guidelines
Local Anaesthesia	• Avoid inferior alveolar nerve block (IANB) unless absolutely necessary - Prefer infiltration or intraligamentary anaesthesia - Avoid epinephrine unless needed - General anaesthesia in hospital is an option
Periodontics	• Emphasize optimal oral hygiene - Use chlorhexidine rinse pre-procedure - No factor replacement needed for scaling/polishing - Factor replacement required for surgery or implants - Use local haemostatic agents

Dental Procedure	Management Guidelines
Oral Surgery	• Highest bleeding risk - Pre-op factor levels should be ≥40–50%, ideally 50–100% - May need postoperative factor replacement (especially 3–5 days post-op) - Use antifibrinolytics and local control - Consult haematologist
Endodontics	• Intraligamentary injections acceptable - Prefer endodontics over extraction - Be cautious with clamp and saliva ejector placement - Some procedures may need factor replacement; consult haematologist
Operative/ Restorative/ Prosthodontics	• Generally safe, no significant bleeding - Careful clamp and ejector use - Ensure prostheses do not traumatize soft tissue
Orthodontics	• No factor replacement needed - Avoid soft tissue trauma from wires

Post-Operative Care

Instructions After Extraction:

- No spitting or straw sucking for 24 hours.

Oral Hygiene:

- Patients may neglect hygiene due to fear of bleeding.
- Emphasize gentle but consistent hygiene.
- For platelet counts <20,000:
    - Modify brushing/flossing techniques.
    - Use chlorhexidine rinses as adjuncts.
- Monitor for periodontal disease.

Dental Management of Patients Taking Anticoagulation Medications

Oral anticoagulant and antiplatelet medications are prescribed to prevent or treat thromboembolic conditions such as Deep Vein Thrombosis, Pulmonary

Embolism, and Atrial Fibrillation, which increase the risk of blood clot formation.

They include:

- Anticoagulants: Warfarin and newer DOACs like Dabigatran, Apixaban, Rivaroxaban, Edoxaban
- Antiplatelet agents: Clopidogrel, Aspirin, etc.

Adverse effect:

- The main concern is prolonged bleeding or bruising, especially during dental procedures.

REMEMBER:

- Do NOT routinely stop these drugs before dental treatment, because discontinuation significantly increases the risk of thromboembolism, stroke, or myocardial infarction.

Dental management approach:

- Most procedures can be safely performed while continuing medication
- Control bleeding with local measures, such as:
  - Mechanical pressure
  - Suturing
  - Hemostatic agents (e.g., Gelfoam®, Surgicel®)
  - Antifibrinolytics like Tranexamic acid

NOTE: The risk of stopping therapy is usually greater than the risk of bleeding, which can be effectively managed locally.

Direct-acting oral anticoagulants (DOACs) such as Dabigatran, Apixaban, Rivaroxaban, and Edoxaban are used to prevent and treat Deep Vein Thrombosis, Pulmonary Embolism, and reduce stroke risk in Atrial Fibrillation.

Key Differences from Warfarin

- Targeted mechanism of action
- Fixed dosing
- Predictable pharmacokinetics
- Shorter half-life
- Minimal monitoring required
- Fewer drug and food interactions

Dental Management – Evidence Summary

- There is no strong high-quality trial evidence, but available data suggest:
    - No need to routinely stop DOACs before most dental procedures
- Guidelines (European Heart Rhythm Association):
    - Safe to continue for:
        - 1–3 tooth extractions
        - Periodontal surgery
        - Abscess incision
        - Implant placement

Systematic Review Findings

- 2019 meta-analysis:
    - No significant difference in bleeding whether DOACs were continued or stopped
    - Evidence quality is low → interpret cautiously
- 2018 review (low–moderate risk procedures):
    - Low-risk: LA, restorations, scaling, single extraction
    - Moderate-risk: 2–4 extractions, minor gingival surgery
    - Bleeding was generally mild and manageable with local measures

Clinical Approach

- Continue DOACs for most procedures
- Use local haemostatic measures for bleeding control
- In higher-risk cases:
    - Consider timing the procedure away from peak drug levels (after last dose)

Warfarin (Vitamin K antagonist)

Evidence-based recommendations:

- Continue warfarin for:
    - Tooth extractions (single or multiple)
    - Minor oral surgery

INR guidelines:

- INR ≤ 3.0 → Safe to proceed
- INR ≤ 3.5 → Safe for uncomplicated extraction
- INR up to 4.0 → Some experts consider acceptable

Important:

- Do NOT aim for subtherapeutic INR → increases thromboembolic risk
- Always check recent INR (within 24–72 hrs)

Antiplatelet Therapy

Includes:

- Aspirin
- Clopidogrel
- Prasugrel
- Ticagrelor
- Ticlopidine

Single or Dual Antiplatelet Therapy (DAPT)

Key recommendations:

- Do NOT discontinue, especially in:
  - Post-stent patients
  - Recent MI
  - High cardiovascular risk

Evidence:

- No significant increase in bleeding vs controls
- Bleeding (if occurs) → manageable with local measures
- No fatal outcomes reported

Strongly emphasize to the patient to:

- Consult cardiologist before stopping
- Premature discontinuation → risk of stent thrombosis (life-threatening)

Safe to proceed without stopping drugs:

- Scaling
- Root planing
- Simple extractions
- Minor oral surgery

Manage bleeding with:

- Pressure packs
- Sutures
- Local haemostatic agents (oxidized cellulose, collagen sponge)
- Tranexamic acid mouthwash

When to be cautious:

- INR > 3.5–4
- Liver disease/coagulopathy

- Multiple extractions + medically complex patient
- Poor local haemostasis expected

When to Activate Emergency Services

- Significant bleeding lasting for hours without clot formation or control after repeated pressure: call emergency services.
- If bleeding stops after pressure within 15-minute intervals: likely manageable without escalation.

Individualize patient management, consult medical specialists when needed, and prioritize risk- benefit analysis before altering anticoagulant/antiplatelet therapy. Keep emergency management tools ready and be proactive in bleeding control measures.

Table 9-3: Anticoagulants & Antiplatelets in Dental Procedures

Feature	**Warfarin**	**Antiplatelets**	**DOACs (Direct Oral Anticoagulants)**
Examples	Warfarin	Aspirin, Clopidogrel, Prasugrel, Ticagrelor, Ticlopidine	Dabigatran, Apixaban, Rivaroxaban, Edoxaban
Mechanism	Vitamin K antagonist	Inhibit platelet aggregation	Direct thrombin or factor Xa inhibitors
Indications	DVT, PE, NVAF, mechanical valves	MI, stroke prevention, post-stent	DVT, PE, NVAF
Monitoring	INR required	Not required	Not required
Pharmacokinetics	Variable	Variable	Predictable, short half-life
Drug/Food Interactions	Many	Few	Few
Evidence Strength	Strong	Strong	Limited

Table 9-4: Dental Management

Aspect	Warfarin	Antiplatelets	DOACs
Routine dental procedures	Continue if INR ≤ 3.0	Continue	Continue
Minor oral surgery	Safe if INR ≤ 3.5–4.0	Continue	Continue (most cases)
Dose alteration needed?	No (if INR controlled)	No	Usually no
Consult physician?	If INR > 4 or high risk	If dual therapy/stent	High-risk cases

Table 9-5: Special Situations

Condition	Recommendation
INR > 4 (Warfarin)	Defer + consult physician
Dual Antiplatelet Therapy (DAPT)	Do NOT stop without cardiologist
Recent Stent/MI	Never discontinue antiplatelets
High bleeding risk surgery	Individualize management
DOACs (if cautious approach)	Schedule at trough/lowest drug level

Note

Some patients who are taking single or multiple anticoagulant medications may have additional co-morbid medical conditions or may be receiving other treatments/medications that can increase the risk of prolonged bleeding after dental treatment, including liver impairment or alcoholism; kidney failure; thrombocytopenia, haemophilia, or other hematologic disorders; or may be currently receiving a course of cytotoxic medication (e.g., cancer chemotherapy). In these situations, it is important to consult the patient's physician and obtain a written consent.

Any suggested modification to the medication regimen prior to dental surgery should be done in consultation with and on advice of the patient's physician only.

References

https://www.ada.org/resources/ada-library/oral-health-topics/oral-anticoagulant-and-antiplatelet-medications-and-dental-procedures

Ardekian, L., Gaspar, R., Peled, M., *et al.* (2000) Does low-dose aspirin therapy complicate oral surgical procedures? *Journal of the American Dental Association*, 131 (3), 331–335.

Balevi, B. (2010) Should warfarin be discontinued before a dental extraction? A decision-tree analysis. *Oral Surgery Oral Medicine Oral Pathology Oral Radiology Endodontology*, 110, 691–697.

Frachon, X., Pommereuil, M., Berthier, A.M., *et al.* (2005) Management options for dental extraction in hemophiliacs: a study of 55 extractions (2000-2002). *Oral Surgery Oral Medicine Oral Pathology Oral Radiology Endodontics*, 99 (3), 270–275.

Gupta, A, Epstein, J.B., & Cabay, R.J. (2007) Bleeding disorders of importance in dental care and related patient management. *Journal of the Canadian Dental Association*, 73, 77–83.

Israels, S., Schwetz, N., Boyar, R., *et al.* (2006) Bleeding disorders: characterization, dental considerations and management. *Journal of the Canadian Dental Association*, 72, 827–840.

Jeske, A. & Suchko, G. (2003) Lack of a scientific basis for routine discontinuation of oral anticoagulation therapy before dental treatment. *Journal of the American Dental Association*, 134, 1492–1497.

Konstantinos, K.C, Lillis, T., Tsirlis, A., *et al.* (2012) Dental management of antiplatelet-receiving patients: is uninterrupted antiplatelet therapy safe? *Angiology*, 63, 245–247.

McBee, W.L. & Koerner, K.R. (2005) Review of hemostatic agents used in dentistry. *Dentistry Today*, 24, 62–65.

Morimoto, Y., Niwa, H., & Minematsu, K. (2009) Hemostatic management for periodontal treatments in patients on oral antithrombotic therapy: a retrospective study. *Oral Surgery Oral Medicine Oral Pathology Oral Radiology Endodontology*, 108, 889–896.

Peisker, A., Raschke, G.F., & Schultze-Mosgau, S. (2013) Management of dental extractions in patients with haemophilia A and B: a report of 58 extractions. *Medicina Oral Patologia Oral y Cirugia Bucal,* 19, e55–e60.

Pototski, M. & Amenabar, J.M. (2007) Dental management of patients receiving anticoagulation or antiplatelet treatment. *Journal of Oral Sciences,* 49, 253–258.

Rada, R.E. (2006) Management of the dental patient on anticoagulant medication. *Dentistry Today,* 125 (8), 58–63.

Sandor, G. (2004) Do patients taking oral anticoagulants need to discontinue their medication before surgical procedures? *Journal of the Canadian Dental Association,* 70, 482–483.

Scully, C. & Wolff, A. (2002) Oral surgery in patients on anticoagulant therapy. *Oral Surgery, Oral Medicine, Oral Pathology, Oral Radiology, Endodontology,* 94, 57–64.

Chapter 10

Dental Management of Pregnant Patients & Those Taking Oral Contraceptives

Introduction

Dental management for pregnant patients emphasizes limiting treatment to periodontal prophylaxis and emergencies, avoiding routine radiographs, and ensuring proper positioning to prevent supine hypotensive syndrome, ideally using the left lateral decubitus position. For patients on oral contraceptives, key considerations include managing exaggerated gingival inflammation, increased risk of dry socket after extractions, and potential reduced effectiveness of birth control if certain antibiotics are prescribed.

DENTAL CARE IN PREGNANCY: KEY GUIDELINES

Timing of Dental Treatment

- First trimester: Highest risk of miscarriage. Avoid elective care; only emergency care if absolutely necessary.
- Second trimester (13–28 weeks): Safest period for elective treatment (e.g., caries, fractured, or abscessed teeth). Most ideal for routine dental procedures.
- Early third trimester: Routine care possible, but monitor comfort.
- Late third trimester: Avoid long appointments; careful positioning required.

Anaesthesia & Medications

- Epinephrine (1:100,000) is safe if intravascular injection is avoided.
- Always weigh benefits vs risks in emergency situations.

Radiographs

- Safe if necessary, using protective measures:
  - Lead apron (thyroid & abdomen).
  - Some obstetricians recommend double aprons.
  - Use digital/E-speed film, rectangular collimation, long cone.
- Pregnant dental staff should also wear aprons.

Positioning

- Second & third trimester: Position on left side (or elevate right hip) to prevent supine hypotensive syndrome (uterus compresses IVC).
- Keep head higher than feet.
- Avoid prolonged supine position (can cause dyspnea, hypotension).

Systemic Concerns

- Hypertension:
  - Mild: ≥140/90 mmHg.
  - Severe: ≥160/110 mmHg. Monitor BP closely.
- Gestational diabetes: Ask about HbA1c and fasting glucose.
- Respiratory changes: Increased rate & dyspnoea; avoid supine position.

Oral Health Considerations

- Scaling & polishing: Safe throughout pregnancy.
- Gingivitis & pyogenic granuloma are common due to elevated oestrogen/ progesterone.
- Emphasize oral hygiene & nutrition education.

Fluoride Supplementation

- If water is not fluoridated, consider 1 mg/day sodium fluoride (3rd–9th month & during breastfeeding).
- Fluoride = Pregnancy Category C → use only with evidence-based justification.

Table 10-1: Denotation of drug categories in pregnancy and breastfeeding

Drug Category	Description	Breastfeeding
A	Controlled studies in women fail to show a risk to the foetus.	Yes
B	Animal or human studies show no significant risk. No controlled studies in pregnant women. Some adverse effects in animals but not confirmed in humans.	Yes
C	No adequate studies in animals or humans, or animal studies show adverse effects but no human data available.	Yes
D	Evidence of foetal risk in humans.	No
X	Studies in animals or humans show definitive foetal risk. Contraindicated in women who are or may become pregnant.	No

Antibiotics in Pregnancy and Nursing

- Safe to prescribe (Category B, minimal foetal risk):
  - Penicillin VK
  - Amoxicillin
  - Clindamycin (recommended if allergic to penicillin)
  - Erythromycin (except *estolate form*, which is hepatotoxic)

- Metronidazole (generally safe after first trimester)
- Azithromycin (Category B)

- To avoid (unsafe/teratogenic):
  - Tetracyclines (tetracycline HCl, doxycycline, minocycline) → Category D
    - Risks: tooth discoloration, inhibition of bone growth in fetus
  - Clarithromycin → Category C
    - Associated with adverse effects in animal studies
- Gestation considerations:
  - Most vulnerable period for teratogenicity: Days 18–60 after conception (organogenesis phase)
  - Physiological changes (↑ blood volume, ↑ renal/hepatic clearance) can alter antibiotic serum levels

Analgesics in Pregnancy and Nursing

- Avoid:
  - Aspirin → risk of delivery complications, maternal postpartum bleeding
  - NSAIDs (ibuprofen, naproxen, etc.):
    - Avoid in first trimester (risk of miscarriage, implantation issues)
    - Avoid in third trimester (risk of premature ductus arteriosus closure, prolonged pregnancy, bleeding)
    - If necessary, only short-term (24–72 hrs) after first trimester
- Safer choices:
  - Acetaminophen (paracetamol) → preferred first-line analgesic during all trimesters and while nursing

Summary of Drugs safety in Pregnancy & Nursing

Table 10-2A: Antibiotics

Drug	FDA Cat.	Pregnancy	Nursing
Amoxicillin	B	Yes	Yes
Penicillin VK	B	Yes	Yes
Erythromycin (except estolate)	B	Yes	Yes
Clarithromycin	C	No	No data (avoid)
Azithromycin	B	Yes (if benefits > risk)	Limited info (caution)
Fluoroquinolones (ciprofloxacin, levofloxacin)	C	No	Discontinue/avoid
Clindamycin	B	Yes (if benefits > risk)	Excreted in milk → caution
Metronidazole	B	Yes (not in 1st trimester)	Stop breastfeeding 12–24h
Tetracyclines	D	No	No

Table 10-2B: Analgesics

Drug	FDA Cat.	Pregnancy	Nursing
Acetaminophen (Paracetamol)	B	Yes	Yes
Aspirin	C/D	Avoid (esp. 3rd trimester)	No
NSAIDs (Ibuprofen, Naproxen, etc.)	B/D	Only after 1st trimester, short-term; avoid in 3rd	No data (effects unknown)
Codeine (with acetaminophen)	C/D	Only if benefit > risk; avoid 3rd trimester	Risk of morphine overdose in baby
Hydrocodone (Vicodin)	C/D	Risk of neonatal resp. depression	Same risk as codeine → avoid

Table 10-2C: Antifungal Agents

Drug	FDA Cat.	Pregnancy	Nursing
Nystatin	B	Yes	Yes
Clotrimazole (topical)	B	Yes	Yes

Table 10-2D: Local Anaesthetics

Drug	FDA Cat.	Pregnancy	Nursing
Lidocaine (with epi)	C	Yes	Yes
Mepivacaine	C	No (fetal bradycardia)	Caution
Bupivacaine	C	No	Yes
Etidocaine, Prilocaine, Articaine	B	Yes	Yes
Benzocaine (topical)	C	No	No

Others:

- Nitrous oxide: *Not classified* – controversial, use only under obstetric consultation.
- Benzodiazepines, barbiturates, triazolam, temazepam: Contraindicated.
- Chlorhexidine oral rinse: Safe.
- Antivirals (acyclovir, valacyclovir, systemic): Generally, not recommended in pregnancy or nursing unless essential.

Oral Contraceptives and Antibiotics

1. General Background

- The interaction between oral contraceptives (OCs) and antibiotics has long been debated.
- The risk of OCs not working is rare, but still possible, especially with low-dose estrogen OCs (<35 μg ethinyl estradiol).

2. Mechanism of Interaction

- Ethinyl estradiol (EE), the oestrogen in OCs:
  - Only 40–50% absorbed systemically in inactive form.
  - Undergoes first-pass metabolism in the liver.
  - Gut flora converts inactive EE into its active form, which is reabsorbed in the intestine.
- Antibiotics (especially broad-spectrum) may disrupt gut flora → reducing reactivation of EE → lowering contraceptive effectiveness.
- Progestins (the other component of OCs) are not affected by gut flora metabolism.

3. Which Antibiotics Are Involved?

- Rifampin (antituberculosis drug) – the most well-documented case of reducing OC effectiveness.
- Other antibiotics (ampicillin, tetracyclines, doxycycline, quinolones, metronidazole, clarithromycin, amoxicillin):
  - Most studies show no significant effect on contraceptive hormone levels.
  - Still, unpredictable individual differences in drug metabolism may increase risk for some women.

4. Clinical Guidelines & Recommendations

- ACOG (American College of Obstetricians & Gynaecologists):
  - Most antibiotics do not significantly reduce OC levels, except rifampin.
- WHO (2004):
  - No significant increase in pregnancy rates among women taking antibiotics + OCs compared to OCs alone.
- ADA Council on Scientific Affairs (2002):
  - Still advises informing women about the possible risk.

5. Practical Advice for Women on OCs Taking Antibiotics

- Use a nonhormonal backup method (e.g., condoms, diaphragm) during antibiotics and for at least 7 days after completing therapy (or until end of cycle, whichever is longer).
- For higher safety:
  - Temporarily switch to a higher-dose OC (with more estrogen + progestin), or
  - Abstain from sexual activity during and after antibiotic course.

Keypoint

While most antibiotics (except rifampin) rarely reduce oral contraceptive effectiveness, the effect cannot be fully ruled out due to individual variability. Therefore, it's safest to recommend backup contraception during and for 7 days after antibiotic use.

References

Amar, S. & Chung, K.M. (1994) Influence of hormonal variation on the periodontium in women. *Periodontology* 2000, 6, 79–87.

American Academy of Pediatric Dentistry (2012). Guideline oral health care for the pregnant adolescent. 35 (6), 150–156.

American Dental Association (2012) Dental Radiographic Examinations: Recommendations for Patient Selection and Limiting Radiation Exposure. www.ada.org/sections/professionalResources/pdfs/Dental_Radiographic_Examinations_2012_pdf [accessed on January 2, 2014].

American Dental Association Council on Scientific Affairs (2002) Antibiotic interference with oral contraceptives. *Journal of the American Dental Association*, 133, 880.

Bauer, K.L. & Wolf, D. (2005) Do antibiotics interfere with the efficacy of oral contraceptives? *The Journal of Family Practice*, 54, 1079–1080.

DeRossi, S.S. & Hersh, E.V. (2002) Antibiotics and oral contraceptives. *Dental Clinics of North America*, 46, 653–654.

Fayans, E.P., Stuart, H.R., Carsten, D. *et al.* (2010). Local anesthetic use in the pregnant and postpartum patient. *Dental Clinics of North America*, 54, 697–713.

Fox, F. (2013) Pregnant dental patients. Health groups spread word that dental care is safe, necessary. *American Dental Association News*, May 20.

Gibson, J. & McGowan, D.A. (1994) Oral contraceptives and antibiotics: important considerations for dental practices. *British Dental Journal*, 177, 419–422.

Giglio, J.A., Lanni, S.M., Laskin, D.M. *et al.* (2009) Oral health for the pregnant patient. *The Journal of the Canadian Dental Association*, 75, 43–48.

Little, J.W., Falace, D.A., Miller, C.S. *et al.* (2008) *Dental Management of the Medically Compromised Patient*, 7th ed., pp. 268–278, 456. CV Mosby, St. Louis.

prevention of dental caries in a group of children. *Oral Implantology*, 4, 23–27.

Michalowicz, B.S., DiAngelis, A.J., Novak, M.J. *et al.* (2008) Examining the safety of dental treatment in pregnant women. *Journal of the American Dental Association*, 139, 686–695.

Moore, P.A. (1998) Selecting drugs for the pregnant dental patient. *Journal of the American Dental Association*, 129, 1281–1286.

Singh, P. (2012) An emphasis on the wide usage and important role of local anesthesia in dentistry: a strategic review. *Journal of Dental Research*, 9, 127–132.

Chapter 11

Dental Management of Patients with Neurological & Psychiatric Disorders

Introduction

Effective dental management for patients with neurological and psychiatric disorders requires a tailored approach incorporating thorough medical history reviews, medication management for side effects like xerostomia, and potential behavioural modifications. Collaboration with psychiatrists and neurologists is essential to coordinate treatment schedules with medication peaks and ensure safety during procedures.

Dental Considerations for Patients with Parkinson's Disease

Parkinson's disease (PD) is a chronic, progressive neurodegenerative disorder caused by degeneration of dopaminergic neurons in the substantia nigra, leading to reduced dopamine levels and characterized pathologically by Lewy bodies (α-synuclein aggregates). It typically affects individuals over 60 years and presents with four cardinal motor features—resting tremor, rigidity, bradykinesia, and postural instability—along with important non-motor symptoms such as dysphagia, cognitive impairment, mood changes, sialorrhea, and autonomic dysfunction (e.g., orthostatic hypotension). Dysphagia is especially common and clinically significant due to aspiration risk, making PD highly relevant in dental care and overall patient management.

Table 11-1: Dental Management of Parkinson's Disease

Category	**Key Points**	**Clinical Tips/Modifications**
1. Pre-consultation Assessment	Confirm stage of PD	Use Hoehn & Yahr (if available)
	Assess wearing-off/OFF periods	Ask timing of last levodopa dose
	Evaluate cognitive status	Simplify instructions and communicate slowly, if impaired
	Assess dysphagia	High aspiration risk, keep HVE ready
	Review medications	Watch for xerostomia, drug interactions
	Involve caregiver	Essential for compliance & history
2. Appointment Scheduling	Short appointments	Prefer ≤ 1 hour
	Timing after medication	60–90 min post-levodopa (ON phase)
	Morning appointments	Less fatigue, better control
	Frequent recalls	Every 3–4 months
	Positioning	Semi-supine to reduce aspiration risk
3. Oral Hygiene Recommendations	Electric toothbrush	Easier with tremors/one-handed use
	Modified handles	Improves grip
	Avoid large-volume rinses	Use gels or supervised rinsing
	Stannous fluoride gel	Prevents root caries
	High-fluoride toothpaste	5000 ppm for high-risk patients

Category	Key Points	Clinical Tips/Modifications
	Xerostomia management	Water, xylitol, saliva substitutes
	Caregiver assistance	Often required daily
4. Challenges During Treatment	Difficulty opening mouth	Use bite block/mouth prop
	Involuntary movements	Treat in ON phase, use 4-handed dentistry
	Tremors/rigidity	Stabilize head, slow movements
	Xerostomia	Affects caries risk & denture retention
	Communication difficulty	Give short, clear instructions
5. Special Considerations	Motor + non-motor symptoms	Include anxiety, depression, cognition
	Orthostatic hypotension	Raise chair slowly
	Prosthodontic issues	Prefer simple, stable designs
	Denture retention problems	Use adhesives, manage dry mouth
	Drug interactions	Avoid dopamine antagonists
	Aspiration risk	Keep High-volume suction ready

Table 11-2: Motor Effects, Oral Complications & Dental Implications in PD

Category	Condition/ Feature	Dental Implications	Clinical Management
Motor-related effects	Dyskinesia (involuntary movements)	Interferes with procedures; jaw/ tongue/lip movements	Short visits; stabilize head/jaw; treat in ON phase
	Bradykinesia	Difficulty opening/ closing mouth; mask-like face	Allow extra time; assist with cheek/lip retraction

(Contd.)

Category	Condition/ Feature	Dental Implications	Clinical Management
	Tremor (pill-rolling)	Poor oral hygiene ability	Educate caregiver; recommend electric toothbrush
	Dystonia	Rigid, painful muscle spasms	May require LA; proceed gently
Other motor/ functional issues	Akathisia (restlessness)	Difficulty sitting still	Secure positioning; schedule during peak medication
	Neck pain	Limited recline tolerance	Maintain ~45° chair position
	Akinesia	Difficulty initiating mouth opening	Use mouth props
	Dysphagia	Aspiration risk; gag reflex	Avoid rinses; minimize water spray; upright position
Oral complications	Sialorrhea (drooling)	Excess saliva pooling; swallowing issue	Frequent suction; medical referral if severe
	Xerostomia	↑ caries risk; poor denture retention	Hydration; fluoride; saliva substitutes; avoid alcohol rinses
Systemic concerns	Orthostatic hypotension	Risk of syncope on position change	Raise chair slowly; avoid sudden movements
	Postural instability	Fall risk	Assist during transfer; avoid leaving patient unattended
	Musculoskeletal pain/ contractures	Poor self-care ability	Caregiver involvement essential
	Cognitive impairment/ depression	Poor compliance; missed instructions	Simplify communication; reinforce instructions
	Urinary urgency	Discomfort during long procedures	Encourage restroom use before appointment

Multiple Sclerosis (MS) – Clinical Synopsis

Multiple sclerosis (MS) is a chronic, immune-mediated, neurodegenerative disease affecting the central nervous system (CNS). It involves destruction of myelin sheaths that insulate nerve fibres in the brain and spinal cord. These demyelinated areas form sclerotic (hardened) plaques, which disrupt normal nerve conduction.

Although the exact cause is unknown, factors likely include:

- Genetic susceptibility
- Autoimmune mechanisms
- Environmental/viral triggers

MS predominantly affects women and typically presents between 20–30 years of age.

Table 11-3: Clinical Features of Multiple Sclerosis

Category	Clinical Features	Key Notes/Relevance
Motor	Spastic paralysis	Increased muscle tone, stiffness
	Muscle weakness (limbs, facial muscles)	Affects mobility and facial function
	Tremors	Impairs coordination and fine movements
	Facial myokymia (twitching)	Characteristic irregular facial movements
	Exaggerated reflexes	Upper motor neuron involvement
Sensory	Paraesthesia	Tingling, numbness (common early symptom)
	Pain (e.g., trigeminal neuralgia)	Severe facial pain; common in MS
Visual	Nystagmus	Involuntary eye movements
	Diplopia (double vision)	Often an early presenting sign
	Visual disturbances	Frequently among first symptoms

(Contd.)

Category	Clinical Features	Key Notes/Relevance
Systemic/ Cognitive	Fatigue	Most common and disabling symptom
	Depression	Affects quality of life and compliance
	Speech disturbance	Slurred or slow speech

Table 11-4: Dental Considerations in Multiple Sclerosis

Category	Feature/Issue	Dental Implications	Clinical Management
Oral manifestations	Trigeminal neuralgia	Severe episodic facial pain	Gentle handling; may need medical/neuro consult
	Facial myokymia	Involuntary facial movements	Can interfere with procedures
	Poor oral hygiene	Due to tremors, spasticity, fatigue	Caregiver support; reinforce hygiene
	Dysarthria/ dysphagia	Difficulty speaking/ swallowing	Aspiration risk; modify procedures
Medication-related	Xerostomia	↑ caries & periodontal disease risk	Hydration, fluoride, saliva substitutes
	Drug side effects	From antispasticity drugs, antidepressants	Review medications before treatment
Appointment considerations	Fatigue/heat sensitivity	Symptoms worsen with stress/ overheating	Short, stress-free appointments
	Morning stiffness	Reduced mobility early in day	Consider afternoon appointments
	Relapse phase	Exacerbation of symptoms	Defer elective dental treatment
Treatment modifications	Local anaesthesia concerns	Interaction with TCAs (epinephrine caution)	Use minimal vasoconstrictor if needed

Category	Feature/Issue	Dental Implications	Clinical Management
	Positioning issues	Neck/head instability	Careful positioning; avoid strain
	Aspiration risk	Due to dysphagia	Upright positioning; suction use
Oral hygiene aids	Limited dexterity	Difficulty brushing/ flossing	Electric toothbrush, floss holders

Table 11-5: Medications for MS – Dental Relevance

Drug Class	Examples	Indication	Dental Implications	Clinical Management
Steroids	Methylprednisolone	Acute exacerbations	Immunosuppression, hyperglycaemia, peptic ulcers, adrenal suppression	Avoid NSAIDs; infection control; consider steroid supplementation for major procedures
Wakefulness Agents	Modafinil	Fatigue	Rash, oral ulcers, dysphagia	Monitor oral lesions; caution if breathing/ swallowing issues
	Amantadine	Fatigue	Xerostomia	Caries prevention, saliva substitutes
K Channel Blocker	Dalfampridine	Improve walking	Dizziness, GI upset	Caution with chair positioning
Muscle Relaxants	Baclofen, Tizanidine, Diazepam	Spasticity	Sedation, hypotension, fatigue	Slow chair movements; post-op caution
Immunosuppressants	Azathioprine, Methotrexate	Suppress T-cells	Anaemia, neutropenia, thrombocytopenia; oral ulcers, candidiasis	CBC monitoring; avoid NSAIDs; infection & bleeding precautions

(Contd.)

Drug Class	Examples	Indication	Dental Implications	Clinical Management
Disease-Modifying Drugs (DMDs)	Interferons, Glatiramer, Natalizumab, Fingolimod, Mitoxantrone, Teriflunomide, Dimethyl fumarate	Relapsing MS	Xerostomia, stomatitis, candidiasis; cytopenias	Monitor CBC; manage oral lesions; frequent recall
Neuropathic Pain Drugs	Gabapentin, Pregabalin, Carbamazepine, Phenytoin	Trigeminal neuralgia	Gingival enlargement (phenytoin); cytopenias (carbamazepine)	Oral hygiene; monitor bleeding/ healing; avoid excess acetaminophen
Anticholinergics	Oxybutynin	Bladder dysfunction	Severe xerostomia → ↑ caries risk	Saliva substitutes; fluoride; frequent recalls

Table 11-6: Dental Treatment Modifications in Multiple Sclerosis

Area	Dental Notes/Problems	Clinical Management
1. Periodontal/ Home Care	Dysphagia, xerostomia, muscle spasticity impair oral hygiene	Caregiver-assisted brushing
	Poor tongue/muscle control	Use electric toothbrush, floss holders, modified handles
	High caries & periodontal risk	Frequent recalls (every 3–4 months)
2. Prosthodontics	Difficulty retaining dentures due to spasticity	Prefer fixed prosthesis when possible
	Poor tolerance to removable prosthesis	Ensure excellent denture fit
	Risk of accidental swallowing	Caregiver instruction essential

Area	Dental Notes/Problems	Clinical Management
	Severe cases	Consider partial dentures over full
3. Dental Caries	Increased caries risk (~21% higher)	Personalized caries management plan
	Xerostomia + poor hygiene	Frequent fluoride application (varnish, gel, toothpaste)
	Dietary factors	Diet counselling (reduce sugar intake)
	Reduced salivary flow	Use salivary substitutes/ stimulants

Epilepsy – Clinical Synopsis

Epilepsy is a chronic neurological condition characterized by recurrent, unprovoked seizures due to abnormal electrical activity in the brain, presenting with manifestations ranging from brief lapses in awareness to generalized convulsions, sometimes accompanied by aura, automatisms, or post-ictal confusion.

From a dental perspective, patients may be on antiepileptic drugs such as Phenytoin, Carbamazepine, or Valproate, which can cause oral side effects like gingival hyperplasia (notably with phenytoin), xerostomia, delayed healing, or thrombocytopenia; dental management requires thorough medical history, identification of seizure triggers (stress, flashing lights), scheduling short morning appointments, ensuring drug compliance, and having emergency preparedness for seizure episodes (positioning patient safely, avoiding restraint, maintaining airway).

Elective procedures should be deferred in poorly controlled cases, and prosthetic or restorative designs should minimize risk of trauma during seizures, making preventive and minimally invasive care particularly important.

Table 11-7: Common oral adverse effects of anti-epileptic drugs

Drug	Key Oral Adverse Effects	Important Clinical Notes
Phenytoin	• Gingival enlargement • Delayed healing • Gingival bleeding	Classic drug causing **gingival hyperplasia** (very common)
Valproic Acid	• Bone marrow suppression • Thrombocytopenia • ↓ Platelet aggregation • Gingival enlargement • Petechiae • Xerostomia	High **bleeding risk** → check platelet count before surgery
Carbamazepine	• Agranulocytosis • (↓ neutrophils) • Aplastic anemia • Xerostomia • Gingival bleeding • Petechiae	Infection risk due to **neutropenia**
Phenobarbital	• Xerostomia • Stomatitis • Drowsiness	CNS depression → caution with sedation
Gabapentin	• Stomatitis • Glossitis • Oral oedema • Dysgeusia	Usually mild, symptomatic management
Lamotrigine	• Stevens–Johnson syndrome • Oral ulcers • Cheilitis	**Medical emergency** if ulcers + skin lesions
Levetiracetam	• Gingivitis • Xerostomia • Stomatitis • Oral/facial oedema	Generally well tolerated

Table 11-8: Common Oral Features in Epileptic Patients

Oral Feature	Description/ Cause	Common Sites	Management	Key Clinical Notes
Drug-Induced Gingival Enlargement	Most commonly due to **Phenytoin**	Anterior labial gingiva (maxillary & mandibular)	• Reinforce meticulous oral hygiene • Scaling & plaque control • Periodontal surgery if severe • Physician consult for drug substitution	Plaque is a major contributing factor; prevention is critical
Oral Soft-Tissue Lacerations	Due to involuntary biting during seizures	Tongue, cheek, lips	• Smooth sharp restorations/ dentures • Wound care • Recommend mouthguard (esp. nocturnal seizures)	Lateral tongue bites are highly suggestive of seizures
Broken Teeth	Trauma or clenching during seizure episodes	Any tooth (often posterior)	• Evaluate for fractures (enamel/dentin/ root) • Manage accordingly (restoration, RCT, etc.) • Preventive mouthguard	Always rule out **cracked tooth syndrome** and root fractures

Key Questions to Ask an Epileptic Patient:

These questions help assess seizure control, safety, and dental risks:

1. When did the last seizure occur?
   - Determines current control and risk during treatment.
2. What precipitates your seizures?
   - Stress, light, sleep deprivation, missed medications, etc.
3. Do you know or feel when you will get a seizure?
   - Some patients have an "aura."
4. Did you acquire any oral cavity injuries previously due to seizures?
   - Tongue biting, fractured teeth indicate severity and frequency.
5. What medications do you take and how regularly do you take them?
   - Check for anti-epileptic drug side effects (gingival enlargement, xerostomia, bleeding).
6. Have seizures affected your mastication and parafunctional habits?
   - Bruxism, clenching, attrition.
7. How frequently do you take oral home care?
   - Important due to xerostomia + gingival enlargement.
8. How frequently do you visit the dentist?
   - Higher recall recommended.

Table 11-9: Dental Concerns in the Epileptic Patient & Management

Category	Clinical Notes/ Concerns	Management	Key Clinical Points
Periodontal Concerns	• Gingivitis & stomatitis (due to drugs like phenytoin, carbamazepine) • Soft-tissue injuries from seizures	• Frequent periodontal maintenance • Reinforce oral hygiene • Manage gingival enlargement (scaling, surgery if needed)	Plaque control is critical to limit drug-induced gingival overgrowth
Prosthetic Concerns	• Risk of trauma from seizures (>1/year) • Fracture of restorations • Dislodgment/ swallowing of removable appliances • Avoid ceramic/ porcelain (fracture risk)	• Prefer fixed prosthesis over removable • Ensure maximum stability if removable used • Night guard for bruxism/nocturnal seizures • Use precision attachments • Reinforce dentures with metal palate/ mesh	Safety priority: prevent aspiration/ swallowing of prosthesis
Operative/ Restorative Concerns	• Increased caries risk (xerostomia) • Attrition/abrasion → material failure risk	• Fluoride therapy, saliva substitutes • Regular recall visits • Rubber dam use recommended • Select strong restorative material (e.g., amalgam in high stress)	Avoid brittle materials in high occlusal load cases

Table 11-10: Dental Drug–Antiepileptic Drug Interactions

1. Valproic Acid/Valproate Sodium

Drug Class	Interacting Drug	Effect	Management
Analgesics/ NSAIDs	Aspirin, NSAIDs	↑ Bleeding, ↑ valproate levels	Avoid high doses; monitor
	Hydrocodone + Ibuprofen	↑ Bleeding + CNS depression	Use with caution
Antibiotics	Erythromycin, Clarithromycin	↑ Valproate levels	Avoid → Use azithromycin
Sedatives	Lorazepam	↑ Benzodiazepine levels → CNS depression	Avoid
	Diazepam, Alprazolam	Additive CNS depression	Use with caution
Other	TCAs	↑ Antidepressant levels	Avoid
	Opioids	↑ CNS depression	Use with caution

2. Carbamazepine

Drug Class	Interacting Drug	Effect	Management
Antifungals	Azoles (fluconazole, ketoconazole)	↑ Carbamazepine, ↓ antifungal	Contraindicated
Analgesics	Acetaminophen	↑ Hepatotoxicity	Avoid
	Diflunisal	↑ SIADH (hyponatremia)	Monitor/avoid
	NSAIDs	↑ SIADH risk	Monitor
Antibiotics	Ciprofloxacin	↑ Carbamazepine levels	Avoid

Drug Class	Interacting Drug	Effect	Management
	Erythromycin, Clarithromycin	↑ Carbamazepine levels	Avoid → Use azithromycin
Opioids	Tramadol	↓ Effect + ↑ seizures + CNS depression	Avoid

3. Gabapentin

Interacting Drug	Effect	Management
Opioids/Codeine combos	↑ CNS depression	Caution
Meperidine	↑ CNS depression	Avoid/caution
Barbiturates	Additive CNS depression	Caution
Benzodiazepines	Additive CNS depression	Caution
Naproxen	↑ Gabapentin levels	Caution
Tramadol	↑ CNS depression + seizures	Avoid

4. Lamotrigine

Interacting Drug	Effect	Management
Phenobarbital	↓ Lamotrigine levels	Monitor/caution

5. Ethosuximide

Drug Class	Interacting Drug	Effect	Management
Antifungals	Azoles	↑ Ethosuximide levels	Monitor/avoid
Antibiotics	Erythromycin, Clarithromycin	↑ Levels	Avoid → Azithromycin
	Ciprofloxacin	↑ Levels	Caution
Sedatives	Benzodiazepines	↑ CNS depression	Caution
Analgesics	Opioids ± NSAIDs	↑ CNS depression	Caution
Other	Tramadol, TCAs	↓ Seizure control + CNS depression	Avoid

6. Phenobarbital

Drug Class	Interacting Drug	Effect	Management
Analgesics	Acetaminophen	↑ Hepatotoxicity	Avoid
	Opioids	↑ CNS + respiratory depression	Caution
Anesthetics	LA + Epinephrine	↑ Methemoglobinemia risk	Avoid
	Benzocaine (topical)	Methemoglobinemia risk	Avoid (esp. infants)
Sedatives	Benzodiazepines	↓ levels but ↑ CNS depression	Caution
	Tramadol	↓ Seizure control	Avoid
Other	Azoles	↓ Antifungal levels	Avoid
	Buspirone	↓ Buspirone levels	Caution
	Corticosteroids	↓ Steroid levels	Caution
	Doxycycline, Metronidazole	↓ Antibiotic levels	Caution

Major Depressive Disorder – Clinical Synopsis and Dental Relevance

Clinical depression is a chronic mood disorder characterized by persistent low mood, anhedonia, fatigue, impaired concentration, sleep and appetite disturbances, and may be associated with psychomotor changes and suicidal ideation; it often involves dysregulation of neurotransmitters such as serotonin and norepinephrine. In dental practice, patients may present with poor oral hygiene, high caries risk, xerostomia (commonly due to antidepressants like Selective Serotonin Reuptake Inhibitors), bruxism, and neglect of dental care. Management requires a compassionate, non-judgmental approach with short, well-structured appointments, reinforcement of oral hygiene, and monitoring for drug interactions (e.g., SSRIs increasing bleeding risk when combined with NSAIDs). Dentists should also be alert to signs of self-neglect or suicidality and coordinate care with mental health professionals when necessary.

Dental Interactions & Side Effects of Antidepressants

Table 11-11: Common Dental Side Effects of Antidepressants

Antidepressant Class	**Dental Effects**
SSRIs/SNRIs/TCAs/MAOIs	Xerostomia → ↑ caries, mucositis, denture sores
TCAs	Orthostatic hypotension (risk during chair position changes)
SSRIs/SNRIs/MAOIs	Increased bleeding tendency (platelet inhibition—mild)
TCAs & tetracyclics, MAOIs	Sedation → ↑ fall risk in dental office
Carbamazepine (when used for depression)	Leukopenia → infection risk *(rare)*

Serotonin Syndrome (Serotonin Toxicity)

Life-threatening → Must be recognized by dentists.

Triad of symptoms:

1. Altered mental status: agitation, confusion
2. Neuromuscular changes: myoclonus, tremor, rigidity
3. Autonomic hyperactivity: fever, tachycardia, diaphoresis

Why important for dentists?

- Triggered by combinations of serotonergic antidepressants + certain dental drugs.

Most risky combinations:

MAOIs (highest risk) +

- Tramadol
- Meperidine
- Fentanyl

- Dextromethorphan
- Sympathomimetics, some decongestants

Avoid these completely in MAOI patients.

SSRIs/SNRIs/TCAs (lower risk, but documented cases) with:

- Tramadol
- Dextromethorphan (in cough syrups)
- Fentanyl
- Meperidine
- Even oxycodone (rare)

Safer opioid choice:

Morphine (non-serotonergic → lowest risk)

Dentist must:

- Avoid interacting drugs
- Warn patient about symptoms
- Refer to emergency service if suspected

References

Becker, D.E. (2008) Psychotropic drugs: implications for dental practice. *Anesthesia Progress*, 55 (3), 89–99.

Buckley, N.A., Dawson, A.H., & Isbister, G.K. (2014) Serotonin syndrome. *British Medical Journal*, 348, g1626.

Desai, J. (2008) Perspectives on interactions between antiepileptic drugs (AEDs) and antimicrobial agents. *Epilepsia*, 49 (Suppl. 6), 47–49.

Eltas, A., Kartalcı, S., Eltas, S.D., *et al.* (2013) An assessment of periodontal health in patients with schizophrenia and taking antipsychotic medication. *International Journal of Dental Hygiene*, 11 (2), 78–83.

Treatment. *American Psychiatric Pub.*

Goulet, J.-P., Perusse, R., & Turcotte, J.-Y. (1992) Contraindications to vasoconstrictors in dentistry: Part III. *Oral Surgery, Oral Medicine, Oral Pathology*, 74, 692–697.

Haas, D.A. (1999) Adverse drug interactions in dental practice: interactions associated with analgesics, Part III in a series. *Journal of the American Dental Association*, 130 (3), 397–407.

Hersh, E.V. (1999) Adverse drug interactions in dental practice: interactions involving antibiotics. Part II of a series. *Journal of the American Dental Association*, 130 (2), 236–251.

Karp, J.M. & Moss, A.J. (2006) Dental treatment of patients with long QT syndrome. *Journal of the American Dental Association*, 137 (5), 630–637.

Keene, J.J., Galasko, G.T., & Land, M.F. (2003) Antidepressant use in psychiatry and medicine: importance for dental practice. *Journal of the American Dental Association*, 134 (1), 71–79.

Lambrecht, T.J., Greuter, C., & Surber, C. (2013) Antidepressants relevant to oral and maxillofacial surgical practice. *Annual of Maxillofacial Surgery*, 3, 160–166.

Mitra, S. & Sinatra, R.S. (2004) Perioperative management of acute pain in the opioid-dependent patient. *Anaesthesiology*, 101 (1), 212–227.

Moore, P.A. (1999) Adverse drug interactions in dental practice: interactions associated with local anesthetics, sedatives and anxiolytics. Part IV of a series. *Journal of the American Dental* 1891–1896.

Tani, H., Uchida, H., Suzuki, T., *et al.* (2012) Dental conditions in inpatients with schizophrenia: a large-scale multi-site survey. *BMC Oral Health*, 12, 32–38.

Wynn, R.L. (1992) Antidepressant medications. *General Dentistry*, 40, 192–197.

Yagiela, J.A. (1999) Adverse drug interactions in dental practice: interactions associated with vasoconstrictors. Part V or a series. *Journal of the American Dental Association*, 130, 701–709.

Yagiela, J.A., Duffin, S.R., & Hunt, L.M. (1985) Drug interactions and vasoconstrictors used in local anesthetic solutions. *Oral Surgery, Oral Medicine, Oral Pathology*, 59, 565–571.

Chapter 12

Dental Management of Patients Undergoing Chemotherapy & Radiotherapy

Introduction

Dental management for patients undergoing chemotherapy and radiotherapy is divided into three critical phases: pre-treatment, during treatment, and post-treatment. The primary goals are to eliminate existing infections, minimize side effects like mucositis and xerostomia, and prevent long-term complications such as osteoradionecrosis (ORN).

Table 12-1: Oral adverse effects after Head & neck radiation or chemotherapy

1. **Hyposalivation (Xerostomia)**

Category	**Subcategory**	**Details/Features**	**Clinical Notes**
Causes	Radiation Therapy (Acute)	Inflammatory reactions → temporary xerostomia	Usually reversible
	Radiation Therapy (Chronic)	Fibrosis, loss of acinar cells, ↓ blood flow	Often permanent damage
	Chemotherapy	Toxic effects on salivary glands	Variable severity
Clinical Features	—	Dry mouth & lips	Common complaint

Category	Subcategory	Details/Features	Clinical Notes
	—	Fissured tongue	Due to dryness
	—	Atrophic filiform papillae	Smooth tongue appearance
Management	Coating Agents	Bismuth salicylate, Sucralfate	Protect mucosa
	Lubrication	Water-soluble lubricants	Symptomatic relief
	Saliva Stimulants	Guaifenesin (200–400 mg, 3–4×/day)	For thick/ropy saliva
		Sugar-free gum/candies, xylitol products	Stimulate salivary flow
	Topical Analgesics	Benzocaine, Lidocaine (viscous)	Short-term relief only
	Oral Hygiene Adjuncts	Moisturizers (Biotène®), alcohol-free rinses (Chlorhexidine), water sips, club soda, ice chips	Maintain oral environment
	Pharmacologic Stimulants	Pilocarpine, Cevimeline	Variable response
	Antifungal Therapy	For Oral Candidiasis	Use topical antifungals

2. Oral Mucositis (Stomatitis)

Category	Subcategory	Details/Features	Clinical Notes
Causes	Chemotherapy	Death of epithelial basal cells	Leads to mucosal breakdown
		Thinning and ulceration of oral epithelium	Painful lesions
		Secondary infection → risk of sepsis	Serious complication
	Radiation	Acute and temporary	Usually reversible

(Contd.)

Category	Subcategory	Details/Features	Clinical Notes
		Initial: white appearance/erythema	Early sign
		Progression → ulceration + pseudomembrane	Advanced stage
Sites	Common Sites	Lips, tongue, floor of mouth, buccal mucosa, soft palate	Frequently involved
	Spared Areas	Hard palate, gingiva	Relatively resistant
Management	Primary Goal	Pain control	Essential for quality of life
	Impact	Difficulty in swallowing, speech, sleep	May cause dehydration & malnutrition
	Nutrition	Nutritional counselling	Critical supportive care
	Oral Hygiene	Brush 2–3×/day (soft brush)	Maintain cleanliness
		Electric toothbrush (with caution)	Avoid trauma
		Non-fluoridated toothpaste	If burning sensation present
		Gentle flossing	Prevent plaque buildup
	Lip Care	Water-soluble jelly	Prevent cracking
	Rinses	Fluoride applications	Caries prevention
		Alcohol-free mouth rinse (Chlorhexidine)	Infection control
		Salt/sodium bicarbonate rinses	Soothing effect

Category	Subcategory	Details/Features	Clinical Notes
		Severe cases: 1:4 hydrogen peroxide (1–2 days) → then saline/ bicarbonate	Short-term debridement
		Ice chips, frequent water rinses	Symptomatic relief
	Analgesics	Lidocaine (viscous 2%)	Pain relief
		Benzocaine 20%/ Orabase®	Local relief
	Coating Agents	Diphenhydramine mixtures	Mucosal protection
	Salivary Support	Xylitol-containing gum	Saliva stimulation
	Systemic Adjunct	Amifostine (IV)	Selected oncology use
Healing	Recovery	Resolves with normalization of WBC count	Linked to immune recovery
	Post-radiation	Healing in 3–6 weeks	Gradual resolution

3. Pain (Neurotoxicity/Nerve Damage)

Causes

- Chemotherapy
  - Tooth pain mimicking toothache
  - Especially with platinum agents and plant alkaloids (e.g., vincristine, vinblastine)
- Radiation & Surgery
  - Tumor invasion of neural tissues
  - Direct neuronal damage

- Secondary factors
    - Tooth hypersensitivity due to:
        - Reduced saliva
        - Lowered salivary pH

Dental Management

- Tooth pain is usually transient
- Often subsides after dose reduction or discontinuation of chemotherapy
- Severe pain is managed by the oncologist with systemic analgesics.

Information to Obtain from the Patient

When interviewing a patient who is about to begin chemotherapy, is currently receiving chemotherapy/radiation, or has received such treatment in the past, the dentist should obtain the following information:

1. Type of cancer diagnosed
2. Presence of any other medical conditions
3. Current or past cancer treatment
    - Radiation therapy
    - Chemotherapy
    - Both radiation and chemotherapy
4. Details of the chemotherapy regimen
    - Name of the drug(s) used
    - Number of cycles completed
    - Route of administration (oral, intravenous, etc.)
5. Current hematologic status
    - White blood cell (WBC) count with differential
    - Platelet count

Treatment Plan for Cancer Patients Receiving Radiation/Chemotherapy Prevention of oral complications associated with high-dose chemotherapy, radiotherapy, or stem-cell transplantation is achieved through regular dental visits and meticulous oral hygiene. Dental management depends on:

- Radiation dose and duration
- Area of the body treated
- Type of cancer therapy
- Presence of treatment-related complications

Pre-radiotherapy/pre-chemotherapy dental screening is critical for optimal cancer care.

Pre-Radiotherapy/Pre-Chemotherapy Dental Preparation

Before cancer therapy begins, the dentist should prepare the patient for anticipated oral complications.

Table 12-2: Pre therapy considerations

Category	Subcategory	Details/Actions	Clinical Notes
Medical Coordination	Oncology Consultation	Coordinate with oncology team	Determine available time for dental care
Medical Evaluation	History & Labs	Review medical history; check WBC, differential, platelets	Assess infection & bleeding risk
Diagnostic Records	Imaging & Models	Full-mouth radiographs, diagnostic casts	Baseline documentation
Dental History & Habits	Oral Hygiene	Assess brushing, flossing, fluoride use	Identify risk factors

(Contd.)

Category	Subcategory	Details/Actions	Clinical Notes
Fluoride Therapy	Indication	Start preventive fluoride before therapy	Reduces radiation caries
	Application Method	Custom trays with full tooth coverage (avoid gingiva)	Begin few days prior
Fluoride Options	Standard Agents	1.1% neutral sodium fluoride (10 min), 0.4% stannous fluoride	Prefer unflavored
	Special Consideration	Use neutral fluoride for porcelain/resin crowns, GIC	Prevent restoration damage
	Contraindicated	Avoid acidulated phosphate fluoride (APF)	Causes tissue irritation
	Alternative	Brush gel for 2–3 min if trays not used	Practical option
Nutritional Assessment	Evaluation	Assess diet & hydration	Prevent dehydration, deficiencies, caries
Radiation Field Assessment	Site-specific Risks	Nasopharynx/ soft palate → xerostomia, caries	Anticipate complications
		Salivary glands → xerostomia, caries	Major salivary impact
		Mandible → osteonecrosis	High-risk bone
Primary Dental Care (Priority)	Infection Control	Treat active infections	Essential before therapy
	Extractions	Remove hopeless teeth	Reduce future complications

Category	Subcategory	Details/Actions	Clinical Notes
	Periodontal Care	Scaling, debridement	Lower infection load
	Irritant Removal	Ill-fitting dentures, orthodontic appliances	Prevent trauma
	Third Molars	Consider extraction (especially partially erupted)	Infection risk
	Timing	Complete extractions ≥7–10 days before therapy	Allow healing time
Secondary Dental Care	Restorative	Treat all caries (including incipient)	Comprehensive care
	Endodontics	Perform RCT where needed	Preserve teeth
	Restorations	Replace faulty restorations	Prevent breakdown
	Prosthodontics	Consultation if required	Functional rehab
Prosthodontic/ Orthodontic Evaluation	Appliance Check	Evaluate all appliances	Ensure safety
	Adjustment	Remove sharp edges/irritants	Prevent mucosal injury

Dental Management During Active Cancer Therapy

During cancer therapy, the primary goals are to maintain optimal oral hygiene and manage oral adverse effects of chemotherapy and/or radiotherapy.

General Principles

- Maintain close and continuous communication with the oncology team
- Prevent oral infections and tissue trauma, which may lead to systemic infection and potentially life-threatening complications.

Table 12-3: Dental Management During Active Cancer Therapy

Category	Subcategory	Details/ Guidelines	Clinical Notes
Medical Coordination	Oncology Consultation	Maintain continuous communication with oncologist	Essential for safe care
	Antibiotic Prophylaxis	Assess need before procedures	Case-dependent decision
Hematologic Status (Chemotherapy)	Lab Monitoring	Check WBC, ANC, platelet count	Always before treatment
	Treatment Delay Criteria	Platelets < 75,000/ mm^3	Risk of bleeding
		ANC < 1,000/mm^3	High infection risk
		Abnormal coagulation factors	Increased bleeding risk
	If Treatment Unavoidable	Discuss antibiotic prophylaxis	Coordinate with oncologist
Central Venous Catheter	Management	Consult oncologist for antibiotic prophylaxis	Prevent catheter-related infections
Dental Visits & Maintenance	Follow-up	Regular dental visits	Increase frequency if symptomatic
	Prevention Focus	Prevent mucositis, infections, trauma	Key during therapy
Extractions During Radiotherapy	Recommendation	Avoid tooth extractions	High-risk period
	Reason	Vascular disruption + radiation damage	Leads to Osteoradionecrosis

Category	Subcategory	Details/ Guidelines	Clinical Notes
Emergency Extractions	Protocol	Antibiotics before & after extraction	Reduce infection risk
	Adjunct	Consider hyperbaric oxygen therapy	Improves healing
	Support	Reinforce oral hygiene	Essential
Timing of Extractions	Pre-Radiotherapy	Wait 14–21 days before starting radiation	Allow healing
	Low Risk Condition	≥21 days healing → minimal risk of ORN	Ideal scenario
	Radiation Dose Factor	<5000 cGy to mandible → lower risk	Dose-dependent
	Post-Radiotherapy	No completely safe time for extraction	Avoid for years
Salivary Changes	Xerostomia	Thick/ropy or reduced saliva	High caries risk
	Prevention	Meticulous oral hygiene	Prevent infection & breakdown
Chemotherapy Considerations	Immunosuppression	Review WBC, ANC, platelets	Defer treatment if low
Oral Hygiene Instructions	Patient Education	Gentle brushing & flossing	Reinforce regularly
Fluoride Therapy	Continuation	Maintain fluoride use during therapy	Prevent radiation caries

After cancer therapy, dental management focuses on maintenance of oral health, early detection of late complications, and long-term monitoring, particularly in patients who received radiation therapy, chemotherapy, or stem-cell transplantation.

Table 12-4: Dental Considerations After Completion of Cancer Therapy

Category	Subcategory	Details/Guidelines	Clinical Notes
Resolution of Oral Complications	Status Assessment	If complications resolved → maintain oral health	Some effects may persist temporarily
Oral Hygiene Maintenance	Home Care	Gentle brushing & flossing	Lifelong adherence essential
Fluoride Therapy	Continuation	Continue fluoride indefinitely	Prevents radiation caries & demineralization
Dental Treatment After Therapy	Eligibility	Treat pending dental issues if patient not immunocompromised	Ensure systemic stability
	High-Risk Patients	Stem-cell transplant, antiresorptive drugs	↑ risk of Osteonecrosis of the Jaw
Post-Radiation Follow-Up	Initial Phase	Every 4–8 weeks for first 6 months	Close monitoring
	Long-Term	Individualized recall schedule	Based on risk
Long-Term Risks	Monitoring	Caries, xerostomia, osteonecrosis	May be permanent
	Xerostomia	Persistent dry mouth	Requires ongoing care
Nutritional Management	Diet	Continue dietary modifications	Prevent deficiencies
	Support	Nutritional supplementation if needed	Coordinate with physician
Prosthodontic Considerations	Existing Dentures	Reevaluate and remove irritants	Prevent mucosal trauma
	Old Dentures	Avoid use	Risk of injury

Category	Subcategory	Details/Guidelines	Clinical Notes
	New Dentures	Delay ≥1 year post-radiation	Allow tissue healing
	Advanced Options	Overdentures, implant-supported dentures	Reduce masticatory load

References

American Academy of Pediatrics (2013) *Guideline on dental management of pediatric patients receiving chemotherapy, hematopoietic cell transplantation, and/or radiation.* http://www.aapd.org/media/Policies_Guidelines/G_Chemo.pdf [accessed on January 13, 2014].

Andrews, N. & Griffiths, C. (2001) Dental complications of head and neck radiotherapy. *Australian Dental Journal*, 46, 174–182.

Atri, R., Dhull, A.K., Dhankhar, R., *et al.* (2007) Orodental care related to radiotherapy for head and neck cancer. *Journal of Oral Health & Community Dentistry* 1, 59–62.

Brosky, M.E. (2007) The role of saliva in oral health: strategies for prevention and management of xerostomia. *The Journal of Supportive Oncology*, 5, 215–225.

Cacchillo, D., Barker, G.J., & Barker, B.F. (1993) Late effects of head and neck radiation therapy and patient/dentist compliance with recommended dental care. *Special Care Dentist*, 13, 159–162.

Carl, W. (1995) Oral complications of local and systemic cancer treatment. *Current Opinion in Oncology*, 7, 320–324.

Chai, W.L., Ngeow, W.C., Ramli, R. *et al.* (2006) Managing complications of radiation therapy in head and neck cancer patients: Part II. Management of radiation-induced caries. *Singapore Dental Journal*, 28, 4–6.

Burket's Oral Medicine, 11th ed, pp. 153–189. BC Decker Inc., Lewiston, NY.

Epstein, J.B. & Huhmann, M.B. (2011b) Dietary and nutritional needs of patients after therapy for head and neck cancer. *Journal of the American Dental Association*, 143, 588–592.

Fleming, P. (1999) Dental management of the paediatric oncology patient. *Current Opinion in Dentistry*, 1, 577–582.

Gerngross, P.J., Martin, C.D., Ball, J.D. *et al.* (2005) Period between completion of radiation therapy and prosthetic rehabilitation in edentulous patients: a retrospective study. *Journal of Prosthodontics*, 14, 110–121.

Hong, C.H., Allred, R., Napenas, J.J. *et al.* (2010) Antibiotic prophylaxis for dental procedures

Jensen, S.B., Pedersen, A.M., Reibel, J. *et al.* (2003) Xerostomia and hypofunction of the salivary glands in cancer therapy. *Support Care Cancer*, 11, 207–225.

National Cancer Institute (2013) *PDQ® Oral complications of chemotherapy and head/neck radiation.* Bethesda, MD: National Cancer Institute. Date last modified August 11, 2013. http://www.cancer.gov/cancertopics/pdq/supportivecare/oralcomplications/HealthProfessional/page4/AllPages [accessed January 10, 2014].

Ngeow, W.C., Chai, W.L., Rahman, R.A., *et al.* (2006c) Managing complications of radiation therapy in head and neck cancer patients: Part VI. Management of opportunistic infections. *Singapore Dental Journal*, 28, 19–21.

Rahman, R., Ngeow, W.C., Chair, W.L. *et al.* (2006) Managing complications of radiation therapy in head and neck cancer patients: Part III. Provision of dentures. *Singapore Dental Journal*, 28, 7–10.

Sonis, S.T. (2004) A biological approach to mucositis. *The Journal of Supportive Oncology*, 2, 21–32.

Toljanic, J.A., Heshmati, R.H., & Bedard, J.F. (2002) Dental follow-up compliance in a population of irradiated head and neck cancer patients. *Oral Surgery Oral Medicine Oral Pathology Oral Radiology Endodontology*, 93, 35–38.

Toth, B.B., Martin, W.W., & Fleming, T.J. (1990) Complications associated with cancer therapy. *Journal of Clinical Periodontology*, 17, 508–515.

Weinberg, M.A., Segelnick, S.L., & Kye, W. (2011) Dental complications of head and neck cancer radiotherapy. *US Pharmacist*, 36 (Oncology Suppl.), 3–7.

Chapter 13

Dental Management of Musculoskeletal and Connective Tissue Disorders

Introduction

Dental management of patients with musculoskeletal and connective tissue disorders requires a comprehensive approach, primarily focusing on maintaining oral hygiene despite physical limitations. Key considerations include managing dry mouth (xerostomia), addressing temporomandibular joint (TMJ) dysfunction, and adjusting treatment plans based on medications like immunosuppressants.

Musculoskeletal disorders comprise diseases of the muscles, joints and bones, autoimmune disorders, and non-autoimmune disorders.

Osteoporosis

Bisphosphonates are prescribed for the treatment and prevention of:

- Corticosteroid-induced osteoporosis
- Postmenopausal osteoporosis
- Hypercalcaemia of malignancy
    - Reduces bone pain and fracture risk
    - Lowers serum calcium levels

- Paget's disease of bone
- Chronic renal disease patients on dialysis
    - Prevents bone fragility

Mechanism of Action

- Bisphosphonates are potent antiresorptive agents

They:

- Inhibit osteoclast-mediated bone resorption
- Reduce bone turnover
- Allow net bone formation

Result:

- Increased bone density
- Prevention of fractures
- Suppression of pathological bone loss

Table 13-1: Dental Management of Patients on Bisphosphonates

Risk Factor	**Details**	**Clinical Notes**
Duration of Oral Therapy	> 3 years	Increased risk
Oral Bisphosphonates	Overall low but present risk	Not negligible
IV Bisphosphonates	Much higher risk	Especially in cancer patients

Risk of Bisphosphonate-Related Osteonecrosis of the Jaw/Medication-Related Osteonecrosis of the Jaw

General Principles

Category	Guideline	Clinical Notes
Preventive Care	Emphasize oral hygiene & regular check-ups	First-line prevention
Surgical Modifications	Conservative, atraumatic technique of extraction	Reduces bone trauma
Infection Control	Strict sterile protocol	Prevents complications
Adjuncts	Use oral disinfectants (e.g., Chlorhexidine)	Reduces microbial load
Coordination	Physician consultation	Essential before invasive care

Patients on Oral Bisphosphonates

a. < 3 Years Therapy

Aspect	Guideline	Clinical Notes
Dental Procedures	Can perform invasive procedures	Routine care acceptable
Precautions	Standard precautions	No major modification needed

b. >3 Years Therapy

Aspect	Guideline	Clinical Notes
Risk Level	Increased risk of Medication-Related Osteonecrosis of the Jaw	Careful evaluation required
Approach	Risk assessment before invasive procedures	Case-by-case decision

CTx (C-terminal Cross-linked Telopeptide) Test

Always check when tooth extraction and/or dental implant is indicated

Parameter	Details	Interpretation
Purpose	Measures bone resorption	Marker of bone turnover
>150 pg/mL	Low risk	Dental procedures generally acceptable
<100 pg/mL	High risk	Increased risk of MRONJ

Table 13-2: Drug Holiday Protocol

Source/Guideline	Recommendation	Clinical Notes/Interpretation
Marx et al.	Stop drug 3 months before and 3 months after invasive dental procedure + use CTX test	Early proposed protocol aimed at reducing risk of medication-related osteonecrosis of the jaw (MRONJ). CTX used as a surrogate marker, but reliability is now questioned. Not universally accepted today.
American Dental Association (ADA, 2011)	Insufficient evidence to support drug holiday	Routine discontinuation not recommended. Emphasis on risk–benefit assessment. Dental treatment should not be unnecessarily delayed.
American Association of Oral and Maxillofacial Surgeons (AAOMS, 2022 update)	Drug holiday may be considered in high-risk cases (after physician consultation)	More nuanced approach: consider duration of therapy (>4 years), comorbidities (diabetes, steroids), and type of drug. Strong emphasis on interdisciplinary decision-making.
Scottish Dental Clinical Effectiveness Programme (SDCEP)	Do NOT routinely stop medication	Focus on atraumatic technique, primary closure, and informed consent. Drug holiday not shown to significantly reduce MRONJ risk.

(Contd.)

Source/Guideline	Recommendation	Clinical Notes/Interpretation
Denosumab-specific consideration	Timing more important than "holiday"	Because of rebound bone turnover, procedures are ideally planned just before next dose (i.e., end of dosing interval), not prolonged discontinuation.

Table 13-3: Patients on IV Bisphosphonates (High MRONJ Risk Group):

Aspect	Guideline	Clinical Notes/Practical Interpretation
Indication	Common in oncology patients (e.g., metastatic cancer, multiple myeloma)	These patients receive high-dose IV bisphosphonates (e.g., zoledronic acid), making them highest risk for MRONJ
Risk Category	Very high risk for MRONJ	Risk significantly higher than oral bisphosphonates; cumulative dose and duration further increase risk
Dental Procedures	Avoid invasive procedures (extractions, implants, bone surgery)	Even minor trauma can precipitate MRONJ; implants are generally contraindicated
Preferred Care	Non-surgical/ conservative management	Endodontic treatment preferred over extraction; smooth sharp edges, adjust prosthesis to avoid trauma
If Procedure Unavoidable	Strict clinical judgment + mandatory physician/oncologist consultation	Evaluate overall prognosis, urgency (e.g., infection, pain), and alternatives before proceeding
Pre-procedure Planning	Comprehensive risk assessment + informed consent	Discuss MRONJ risk explicitly; document consent carefully
Surgical Approach (if needed)	Atraumatic technique + primary closure	Minimal flap reflection, smooth bone, tension-free closure to reduce exposure risk

Aspect	Guideline	Clinical Notes/Practical Interpretation
Antibiotic Protocol	Consider prophylactic antibiotics	Not universally standardized, but often recommended in high-risk cases
Drug Holiday	Generally, NOT effective for IV bisphosphonates	Long half-life in bone (years); stopping drug does not significantly reduce risk
Post-op Care	Close follow-up + chlorhexidine rinses	Early detection of delayed healing or exposed bone is critical
Implants	**Contraindicated in most cases**	Exception only in rare, carefully selected cases with specialist input

Patients on long-term bisphosphonate therapy, especially IV formulations, must be managed cautiously with emphasis on prevention, conservative treatment, and interdisciplinary consultation.

Osteoarthiritis

Dental management:

1. A medical consultation is usually not required.
2. No antibiotic prophylaxis is required.
3. Keep short appointments due to pain in joints.
4. Semi-supine position in the dental chair may be more comfortable than supine. Patients may require help getting in and out of the chair. Many patients may be using a cane, walker, or a wheelchair.
5. For osteoarthritis of the hand, oral home care devices may need changes: electric toothbrush, bigger handles for toothbrush, and electric flosser.
6. Patients may be taking aspirin or NSAIDs. No contraindications for treatment. May experience slightly more bleeding during a dental procedure (e.g., scaling/root planing, periodontal and implant surgery, and extractions). Symptom management is considered the first-level therapeutic approach.

Rheumatoid Arthiritis

Dental Management:

1. Medical consultation
   - Always consult the physician/rheumatologist to determine active vs-controlled RA.
2. Appointment timing
   - Schedule morning or early afternoon appointments (less fatigue, better joint mobility).
3. Clinical suspicion of RA
   - Suspect RA if patient reports:
     - Polyarthritis
     - Morning stiffness and pain ≥30 minutes
   - Differential diagnosis: Systemic lupus erythematosus (SLE).
4. DMARD therapy
   - Patients on DMARDs are routinely monitored for:
     - Drug toxicity
     - Disease activity
   - Ask patients about their monitoring schedule and recent labs.
5. Rituximab
   - Risk of:
     - Serious infections
     - Delayed wound healing after invasive dental procedures
   - Mandatory consultation with rheumatologist before surgery.
6. Oral health monitoring
   - Monitor:
     - Oral hygiene

  - Caries
  - Periodontal disease

- RA patients have a higher prevalence of periodontal disease.

7. Smoking cessation
   - Tobacco use is a risk factor for RA and worsens disease severity.
8. Corticosteroid therapy
   - Patients on long-term steroids may require stress-dose supplementation for invasive procedures.
   - Always consult the physician.
9. Adverse effects of DMARDs
   - Be alert for:
     - Thrombocytopenia → bleeding risk
     - Leukopenia → increased infection risk
10. Antibiotic prophylaxis
    - Some patients may require prophylaxis depending on immune status.
    - Decision should be made in consultation with physician.
11. Liver function considerations
    - DMARDs can alter liver function tests
    - Antibiotic dose or interval adjustment may be required.
12. TMJ evaluation
    - TMJ involvement is common in RA
    - Anterior open bite may develop due to condylar resorption.
13. Important dental drug interaction
    - Amoxicillin + Methotrexate
      - High-dose amoxicillin can ↑ serum methotrexate levels

Leads to:

- Nausea, vomiting
- Oral ulcers
- Bone marrow suppression → anaemia, bleeding, infections.

Table 13-4: Rheumatoid arthritis Drugs and Dental Implications

Drug Category	Examples	Dental Implications
NSAIDs	Ibuprofen, Naproxen, etc.	Antiplatelet effect → increased bleeding risk during dental procedures
Corticosteroids (oral/ intra-articular)	Prednisone, etc.	May require stress-dose steroid supplementation for invasive dental surgery; depends on daily vs alternate-day dosing
Non-biologic DMARDs	Methotrexate, Hydroxychloroquine, Leflunomide, Sulfasalazine	Immunosuppression → infection risk, bleeding, altered liver function
Methotrexate	Rheumatrex	Stomatitis, oral ulcers (dose dependent); ↑ infection risk; usually continued during dental surgery; MTX + NSAIDs → ↑ MTX toxicity
Hydroxychloroquine	Plaquenil	May cause lichenoid-like oral reactions or rash
Biologic DMARDs (TNF inhibitors)	Adalimumab, Etanercept, Infliximab, Abatacept	↑ risk of infections; recommended to discontinue before surgery and restart after complete wound healing
Rituximab	Rituxan	Severe oral ulcers, cytopenias → infection, bleeding, delayed healing; complete dental care before therapy; invasive dental surgery ≥6 months after last infusion; consult rheumatologist

Drug Category	Examples	Dental Implications
Immunosuppressants (also post-transplant/ IBD)	Azathioprine, Cyclosporine, Tacrolimus	Gingival enlargement (cyclosporine, tacrolimus); difficult oral hygiene; frequent recalls needed
Drug interaction (important)	Cyclosporine + NSAIDs	Increased nephrotoxicity
Immunomodulator	Iguratimod	Elevated liver enzymes; thrombocytopenia
JAK inhibitors	Tofacitinib	Opportunistic infections, ↓ neutrophils, ↑ liver enzymes, nasopharyngitis

Table 13-5: Drug Management Before Dental Extraction & Implants

Drug Category	Examples	Extraction (Minor Oral Surgery)	Implants/Major Surgery	Key Dental Notes
NSAIDs	Ibuprofen, Naproxen	Continue	Continue	Mild ↑ bleeding; avoid prolonged use with methotrexate
Methotrexate	Rheumatrex	Continue	Continue (most cases)	Avoid NSAIDs; monitor for ulcers, infection
Hydroxychloroquine	Plaquenil	Continue	Continue	Very safe; rare lichenoid reactions
Other DMARDs	Leflunomide, Sulfasalazine	Continue	Usually continue	Check CBC/LFT if extensive surgery
Corticosteroids	Prednisone	Continue (no abrupt stop)	Continue + consider **stress dose**	Risk of adrenal suppression, delayed healing
Biologic DMARDs (TNF- inhibitors)	Adalimumab, Etanercept, Infliximab	Usually continue for minor procedures	**Hold (1 dosing cycle prior)**	Restart after complete healing

(Contd.)

Drug Category	Examples	Extraction (Minor Oral Surgery)	Implants/Major Surgery	Key Dental Notes
JAK inhibitors	Tofacitinib	Usually continue	**Hold 3–7 days prior**	Infection risk, neutropenia
Rituximab	Rituxan	Avoid if possible	**Defer surgery** (≥6 months after infusion)	Severe immunosuppression, cytopenias
Immunosuppressants	Azathioprine, Cyclosporine, Tacrolimus	Continue with caution	Continue (physician consult)	Gingival overgrowth; infection risk; avoid NSAIDs with cyclosporine
Iguratimod	Iguratimod	Continue if labs normal	Consider hold if thrombocytopenia	Monitor platelets, liver enzymes

Fibromyalgia

Dental Considerations in Fibromyalgia Patients

1. When fibromyalgia is diagnosed after ruling out all other diseases, no medical consultation is required.
2. If the patient is taking a tricyclic antidepressant (e.g., amitriptyline), limit 1:80,000 epinephrine to a maximum of two cartridges.
3. Xerostomia is a known adverse effect of cyclobenzaprine and pregabalin.
4. Patients with fibromyalgia may present with xerostomia and temporomandibular disorders (TMD); manage appropriately.
5. Due to jaw muscle fatigue, patients may have difficulty keeping the mouth open; use mouth props if necessary.
6. Palpation of head and neck muscular structures should be performed during examination.
7. There is a high prevalence of orofacial pain complaints in patients with fibromyalgia.

Table 13-6: Dental Drug–Fibromyalgia Drug Interactions

Dental Drugs	**Fibromyalgia Drugs**	**Notes/Dental Implications**
Epinephrine	Tricyclic antidepressants (e.g., amitriptyline)	Moderate interaction. Limit epinephrine to 1:100,000, max 2 cartridges (1.7 ml each). TCAs inhibit NE/EPI reuptake → ↑ epinephrine levels → possible cardiac complications. No interaction with SSRIs (e.g., fluoxetine).
Epinephrine	Duloxetine	Moderate interaction. Duloxetine (SNRI) inhibits NE/EPI reuptake → ↑ cardiovascular risk with epinephrine. Limit epinephrine to 1:100,000, max 2 cartridges.
Acetaminophen, codeine, oxycodone, hydrocodone, ibuprofen	Tramadol	Major interaction. Consult physician. ↑ risk of seizures and respiratory depression.
Ciprofloxacin, levofloxacin	Tramadol	Major interaction. Consult physician. May cause seizures.
Lidocaine with epinephrine (dental anesthesia)	Tramadol	Major interaction. Increased seizure risk, especially in elderly, alcohol users/withdrawal, or patients with history of seizures, brain tumor, or head trauma.

Sjogren's Syndrome

Table 13-7: Oral symptoms and dental management

Oral Signs/ Symptoms	Dental Management
Xerostomia and salivary gland hyposalivation	Highly recommended drugs are systemic sialogogues (muscarinic agonists): pilocarpine 5–10 mg three times daily or cevimeline 30 mg three times daily. These agents may not be effective in later stages of SS with irreversible salivary gland damage. Clinical trials show that salivary lubricants and substitutes in severe cases are not clearly agreed upon, though topical moisturizers appear marginally acceptable. Remineralizing products, Oral Biotène products, carboxymethylcellulose or hydroxyethyl solutions, xylitol-containing chewing gum, frequent water intake, and regular oral home care are recommended.
Dysphagia	Clinical studies show promising positive results with electric stimulators.
Oral burning	According to many clinical studies, oral burning is difficult to treat with predictable outcomes; tricyclic antidepressants have been reported to be helpful.
Oral candidiasis *(secondary to oral dryness and/or changes in salivary composition)*	Due to a high rate of resistance to most topical agents, systemic antifungal therapy (fluconazole) is recommended.

<table>
<tr><td>Drugs for SS</td><td>Notes</td></tr>
<tr><td>Treating systemic involvement of SS:
• Infliximab
• Interferon-
• Rituximab</td><td>There is insufficient evidence to routinely prescribe immunomodulators, biologic agents, or monoclonal antibodies, or immunosuppressive drugs for purely oral/oral-symptom control. These drugs may be recommended for systemic SS features including renal, respiratory, hepatic, neurologic, and vascular involvement. Rituximab adverse effects include skin and mouth reactions ranging from Stevens–Johnson syndrome/toxic epidermal necrolysis, increased risk of postoperative infections, and delayed wound healing.
Dental considerations:
• Consult the patient's rheumatologist before dental surgery.
• Use caution when scheduling dental procedures in patients receiving rituximab.
• Some sources recommend a minimum 6-month interval between rituximab infusion and invasive dental surgery (decision depends on indication).
• Consult the treating physician regarding timing of dental surgery.
• Rituximab may cause reactivation of hepatitis B infection.</td></tr>
<tr><td>Treating eye problems</td><td>Artificial tear substitutes, eye ointments or gels, and cyclosporine eye drops (increase tear production).</td></tr>
</table>

Dental Considerations in Sjogren's Syndrome:

Recommend physician consultation to determine whether systemic involvement is present.

1. Review oral symptoms and all current medications the patient is taking.
2. Hyposalivation may lead to dental caries, fungal infections, and periodontal disease, and can significantly affect patient comfort. Encourage regular oral self-examinations to report ulcers or other oral problems. Fluoride supplementation is recommended for high–dental risk patients. Emphasize meticulous home care and frequent recare appointments .
3. Advise patients not to sleep with dentures.

References

American Dental Association Council on Scientific Affairs (2006) Dental management of patients receiving oral bisphosphonate therapy. *Journal of the American Dental Association*, 137 (8), 1144–1150.

Balasubramaniam, R., Laudenbach, J.M., & Stoopler, E.T. (2007) Fibromyalgia: an update for oral health care providers. *Oral Surgery, Oral Medicine, Oral Pathology, Oral Radiology and Endodontology*, 104, 589–602.

Carr, A.J., Ng, W.F., Figueiredo, F. *et al.* (2012) Sjogren's syndrome—an update for dental practitioners. *British Dental Journal*, 213 (7), 353–357.

De Silva, L.A., Kazyiama, H.H., de Siqueira, J.T., *et al.* (2012) High prevalence of orofacial complains in patients with fibromyalgia: a case-control study. *Oral Surgery, Oral Medicine, Oral Pathology, Oral Radiology and Endodontology*, 113, e29–e34.

Edwards, B.J., Hellstein, J.W., & Jacobson, P.L. (2008) Updated recommendations for managing the care of patients receiving oral bisphosphonate therapy: an advisory statement from the American Dental Association Council on Scientific Affairs. *Journal of the American Dental Association*, 139, 1674–1677.

Fleisher, K.E., Welch, G., Kottal, S., *et al.* (2010) Predicting risk for bisphosphonate-related osteonecrosis of the jaws: CTX versus radiographic markers. *Oral Medicine, Oral Pathology, Oral Radiology and Endodontology*, 110 (4), 509–516.

Fugazzotto, P.A., Lightfoot, W.S., Jaffin, R. *et al.* (2007) Implant placement with or without simultaneous tooth extraction in patients taking oral bisphosphonates: postoperative healing, early follow up, and the incidence of complications in two private practices. *Journal of Periodontology*, 7819, 1664–1669.

Grant, B.T., Amenedo, C., Freeman, K., *et al.* (2008). Outcomes of placing dental implants in patients taking oral bisphosphonates: a review of its cases. *Journal of Oral and Maxillofacial Surgery*, 66, 223–230.

Marx, R.E. 2007. *Oral and Intravenous Bisphosphonate-Induced Osteonecrosis of the Jaws: History, Etiology, Prevention, and Treatment*, p. 15. Quintessence, Chicago, IL.

Marx, R.E., Sawatari, Y., Fortin, M. *et al.* (2005). Bisphosphonate-induced exposed bone (osteonecrosis/osteoporosis) of the jaws: risk factors, recognition, prevention, and treatment. *Journal of Oral and Maxillofacial Surgery*, 63, 1567–1575.

Mercardo, R.B., Marshall, R.I., Klestov, A.C., *et al.* (2001) Relationship between rheumatoid arthritis and periodontitis. *Journal of Periodontology*, 72, 779–787.

Migliorati, C.A., Saunders, D., Conlon, M.S., *et al.* (2013) Assessing the association between bisphosphonate exposure and delayed mucosal healing after tooth extraction. *Journal of the American Dental Association*, 144 (4), 406–414.

Otomo-Corgel, J. (2007) Implants and oral bisphosphonates: risky business? *Journal of Periodontology*, 78, 373–376.

Pinto, A. (2014) Management of xerostomia and other complications of Sjogren's syndrome. *Oral Maxillofacial Surgery Clinics*, 26 (1), 63–73.

Rhodus, N.L., Fricton, J., Carlson, P., *et al.* (2003) Oral symptoms associated with fibromyalgia syndrome. *The Journal of Rheumatology* 30, 1841–1845.

Treister, N. & Glick M. (1999) Rheumatoid arthritis: a review and suggested dental care considerations. *Journal of the American Dental Association*, 130, 689–698.

Wang, H. L., Weber, D., & McCauley, L.K. (2007) Effect of long-term oral bisphosphonates on implant wound healing: literature review and a case report. *Journal of Periodontology*, 78, 584–594.

Wu, A.J. (2008) Optimizing dry mouth treatment for individuals with Sjögren's syndrome. *Rheumatic Disease Clinics of North America*, 34 (4), 1001–1010.

Zak, M., Spina, A.N., Spinazze, R.P., *et al.* (2007). Bisphosphonates and the dental patient: Part 1. *Compendium* 28 (9), 510–516.

Chapter 14

Clinical Scenarios

Case 1

61-year-old, male patient.

Patient has the following medical history

Renal allograft recipient (renal transplant done 3 years back), Hypertension, Diabetes Mellitus, hypercholestreamia, Fungal sinusitis and retinitis, on medications.

Noteworthy medications:

Methylprednisolone, Tacrolimus

Chief complaint: Broken maxillary premolar tooth, requiring extraction.

Risk factors

Category	Details
Immunosuppression	Due to Tacrolimus + Methylprednisolone • ↑ Post-op infection • Delayed healing • Opportunistic infections (take fungal infection history)

Category	Details
Diabetes Mellitus	• Impaired wound healing • ↑ Infection risk • Maintain RBS < 180 mg/dL
Renal Transplant Status	• Drug interactions • Nephrotoxicity risk • Graft protection essential
Hypertension	• Stress-induced BP spikes • Vasoconstrictor caution
Steroid Therapy	• Adrenal suppression risk • Consider stress-dose steroids

Pre – Operative protocol

Step	Details
Medical Consultation (MANDATORY)	Written clearance from nephrologist regarding: • Fitness for extraction • Antibiotic prophylaxis need • Steroid supplementation
Investigations	• Renal function tests (Serum creatinine) • HbA1c & RBS • CBC (WBC count)
Drug Considerations	Avoid nephrotoxic drugs: • NSAIDs (diclofenac, high-dose ibuprofen) • Aminoglycosides
Antibiotic Prophylaxis	• Recommended due to immunosuppression • Amoxicillin (if no allergy) • Alternative if required (Clindamycin or Azithromycin)

Operative Protocol

Aspect	Guideline
Glycaemic Control	• Short, Morning appointment • Ensure patient has eaten & taken medications
Local Anaesthesia	• Lignocaine with adrenaline (1:100,000) cautiously • Avoid excess vasoconstrictor
Extraction Technique	• Atraumatic extraction • Minimize tissue injury • Ensure complete curettage & no residual infection • Give sutures • Consider LASER photobiomodulation (if available)
Infection Control	• Strict asepsis • Chlorhexidine pre-rinse

Post operative protocol

Aspect	Guideline
Antibiotics	Continue 5–7 days (as prescribed)
Analgesics	Preferred: Paracetamol, Avoid NSAIDs
Healing Monitoring	Watch for: • Delayed healing • Dry socket • Secondary infection
Steroid Cover	• Consider supplemental dose if on long-term steroids (physician-guided)

Case 2

65-year-old, male patient.

Patient has the following medical history

Liver transplant done 2 months, Hypertension, Diabetes Mellitus (under control) on medications.

Noteworthy medications: Cyclosporine, Steroids

Chief complaint: Grossly carious maxillary molar tooth, requiring extraction.

Risk factors

Risk Factor	Implication in Dental Treatment
Recent liver transplant (2 months)	High infection risk, delayed healing
Immunosuppressive therapy	Opportunistic infections, poor wound healing
Liver function	Possible bleeding tendency
Diabetes	Delayed healing, infection risk
Hypertension	Stress-related complications

Pre Operative protocol

Step	Details
Medical Consultation (MANDATORY)	Written clearance from hepatologist regarding: • Fitness for extraction • Antibiotic prophylaxis need
Investigations	CBC PT/INR For Bleeding risk Blood sugar (HbA1c & RBS) for Glycemic control LFT (if advised) Liver status
Drug Considerations	Avoid: • NSAIDs (diclofenac, high-dose ibuprofen) – Use paracetamol • Aminoglycosides
Antibiotic Prophylaxis	• Recommended due to immunosuppression • Amoxicillin (if no allergy) • Alternative if required (Clindamycin or Azithromycin)

Operative protocol

Aspect	Guideline
Glycemic Control	• Short, Morning appointment • Ensure patient has eaten & taken medications
Local Anesthesia	• Lignocaine with adrenaline (1:100,000) cautiously • Avoid excess vasoconstrictor
Extraction Technique	• Atraumatic extraction • Minimize tissue injury • Ensure complete curettage & no residual infection • Give sutures, use pressure pack, local haemostatic agents • Consider LASER photobiomodulation (if available)
Infection Control	• Strict asepsis and chlorhexidine pre rinse

Post operative protocol

Aspect	Guideline
Antibiotics	Continue 5–7 days (as prescribed)
Analgesics	Preferred: Paracetamol, Avoid NSAIDs
Healing Monitoring	Watch for: • Delayed healing • Dry socket • Secondary infection

Red Flags/Contraindications

Finding	Action
INR > 3	Defer treatment
Uncontrolled diabetes	Postpone
Active systemic infection	Defer
No physician approval	Do NOT proceed

Case 3

65 year old, male patient.

Patient has the following medical history:

Type 2 Diabetes Mellitus (poorly controlled, HbA1c 9%), Hypertension, On aspirin (75 mg daily)

Chief complaint: Multiple Grossly carious teeth in both the arches, requiring extraction and replacement with removable/fixed teeth.

Concerns

- Poor wound healing
- Increased infection risk
- Bleeding tendency (aspirin)
- Risk of hypertensive crisis

Management

- Check blood glucose (preferably <200 mg/dL before procedure)
- Schedule morning appointment
- Do not stop aspirin (minor oral surgery usually safe)
- Use local hemostatic measures, give sutures
- Prescribe prophylactic antibiotics if infection risk high
- Monitor BP before procedure

Case 4

30 year old, female patient

Patient has the following medical history:

- Bronchial Asthma
- Generalized Anxiety Disorder

Chief complaint: Pain in lower left molar tooth requiring Root canal treatment

Key Considerations

Category	Considerations/Management
Patient Conditions	Bronchial Asthma + Generalized Anxiety Disorder
Major Risks	Asthma attack, panic attack, hyperventilation, increased stress response
History to Ask	Last asthma attack, triggers, hospitalization history, current medications, inhaler use
Appointment Planning	Morning appointment, short duration, stress-free environment
Pre-medication	Mild anxiolytic (e.g., benzodiazepine if required)
Inhaler Precaution	Patient must carry salbutamol inhaler; keep accessible chairside
Anxiety Control	Tell-show-do, reassurance, good communication
Sedation Option	Nitrous oxide sedation (safe and effective)
Positioning	Semi-supine (avoid full supine if breathing discomfort)
Local Anaesthesia	Lidocaine with minimal adrenaline; avoid excess vasoconstrictor
Materials to Avoid	Strong odours (eugenol, acrylics), potential irritants
Isolation	Rubber dam preferred (reduces aerosol and aspiration risk)
Intra-op Monitoring	Watch for wheezing, breathlessness, restlessness
Asthma Attack Management	Stop treatment, upright position, salbutamol inhaler (2 puffs), oxygen
Anxiety/Panic Attack	Reassure, slow breathing, pause/terminate procedure if needed

Category	Considerations/Management
Analgesics	Paracetamol preferred; avoid NSAIDs in sensitive patients
Antibiotics	Amoxicillin (if indicated)
Post-op Advice	Stress reduction, continue inhaler, follow-up scheduling

Case 5

50 year old, female patient

Patient has the following medical history:

- Known case of Hyperthyroidism
- History of Atrial Fibrillation

Medications:

- Antithyroid drugs (Carbimazole)
- Beta-blockers (Propranolol)
- Anticoagulants (Apixaban)

Chief complaint: Extraction and replacement with implant of a grossly decayed lower molar tooth.

Key considerations

Category	Findings/Considerations	Dental Management
Medical Conditions	Hyperthyroidism + Atrial Fibrillation	Increased metabolic rate + arrhythmia risk
Common Medications	Antithyroid drugs, Beta-blockers, Anticoagulants	Watch for bleeding & drug interactions
Main Risks	Thyroid storm, tachyarrhythmia, embolism, bleeding	Careful planning required

(Contd.)

Category	Findings/Considerations	Dental Management
Pre-op Evaluation	TSH, T3, T4; Pulse, BP; INR (if warfarin)	Ensure controlled thyroid & stable AF
Need for Consultation	If uncontrolled thyroid or unstable AF	Physician/cardiologist clearance
When to Postpone	Tachycardia (>100 bpm), symptomatic AF, thyrotoxicosis	Defer elective extraction
Local Anaesthesia	Avoid/limit epinephrine (≤0.04 mg)	Prefer plain lignocaine
Stress Reduction	Anxiety may trigger arrhythmia or thyroid storm	Short morning appointment, sedation if needed
Bleeding Risk	Due to anticoagulants	Local haemostatic measures (pressure, sutures)
Intra-op Monitoring	Pulse, signs of distress	Stop if palpitations/ dizziness occur
Post-op Analgesics	NSAIDs increase bleeding risk	Prefer paracetamol
Post-op Advice	Risk of delayed bleeding	Clear instructions + follow-up

Case 6

68 year old female patient with:

- Rheumatoid Arthritis (on methotrexate and steroids)
- Type 2 Diabetes Mellitus (HbA1c = 8%)
- History of Coronary Stent Placement (on dual antiplatelet therapy – aspirin + clopidogrel)

Chief complaint: Extraction and replacement with implant of a grossly decayed lower molar tooth.

Key considerations

Aspect	Rheumatoid Arthritis	Diabetes Mellitus	Cardiac Stent (DAPT)	Overall Clinical Decision
Condition	Rheumatoid Arthritis	Type 2 Diabetes Mellitus	Coronary Stent Placement	Multi-system high-risk patient
Major Risks	Immunosuppression, poor healing, TMJ limitation	Infection, delayed healing, implant failure	Stent thrombosis, bleeding risk	Cardiac risk > others
Drugs	Methotrexate, steroids	Insulin/OHAs	Aspirin + Clopidogrel	Drug interactions critical
Pre-op Assessment	Check steroid use, mouth opening	HbA1c (<7 ideal), FBS	Time since stent, cardiology consult	Prioritize cardiac stability
Can we STOP meds?	Usually continue	Continue	Do NOT stop antiplatelets	Never stop without cardiologist
Appointment Planning	Short visits, joint support	Morning, after meals	Stress reduction	Combine all precautions
Local Anesthesia	No major issue	Avoid infection	Limit epinephrine (≤0.04 mg)	Careful LA use
Bleeding Risk	Mild (if on meds)	Normal/slightly ↑	HIGH (due to DAPT)	Manage locally, not systemically
Bleeding Control	Standard	Standard	Sutures, pressure, tranexamic acid	Key step in extraction
Infection Risk	↑ (immunosuppressed)	↑↑ infection risk	Normal	Consider antibiotics

(Contd.)

Aspect	Rheumatoid Arthritis	Diabetes Mellitus	Cardiac Stent (DAPT)	Overall Clinical Decision
Analgesics	Avoid NSAIDs (if GI/ steroids)	Avoid NSAIDs (renal risk)	Avoid NSAIDs (cardiac)	Prefer paracetamol
Steroid Cover	May be needed	—	—	If long-term steroid use
Extraction	Possible with care	With controlled sugar	Without stopping DAPT	SAFE with precautions
Implants	Delay (healing issues)	Delay if HbA1c >7	Delay if recent stent	Postpone initially
Ideal Implant Timing	Stable disease	HbA1c <7%	After cardiologist clearance	Only after stabilization
Emergency Risk	Adrenal crisis (rare)	Hypo/ hyperglycaemia	Angina/MI	Be fully prepared

www.ingramcontent.com/pod-product-compliance
Lightning Source LLC
LaVergne TN
LVHW090408210926
848480LV00002B/494

* 9 7 9 8 9 0 4 7 9 6 0 4 4 *